Super Simple Air Fryer Dishes

A Collection of Simple and Delicious Air Fryer Recipes

By Samantha Hendrick

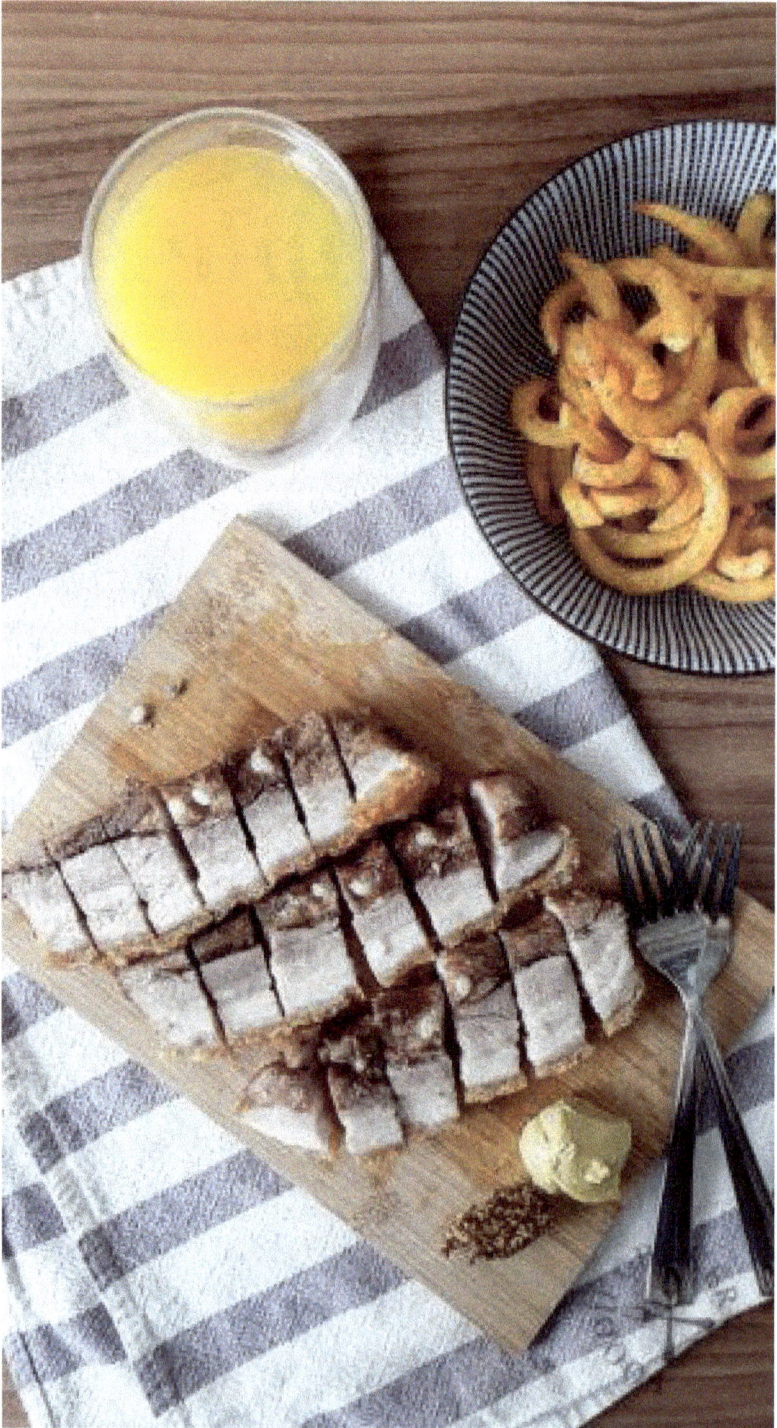

Table of Contents

Grilled Thighs with Honey Balsamic Sauce

Servings per Recipe: 8

Cooking Time: 40 minutes

Ingredients:

- 1/3 cup honey /83ML
- 2 tablespoons balsamic vinegar /30ML
- 2 tablespoons butter /30G
- 3 cloves of garlic, minced
- 8 bone-in chicken thighs
- Chopped chives for garnish
- Lemon wedges for garnish
- Salt and pepper to taste

Instructions:

1) Season the chicken with salt and pepper to taste. Add the butter, balsamic vinegar, honey, and garlic. Allow to marinate for 120 minutes inside the fridge.
2) Preheat mid-air fryer to 390° F or 199°C .
3) Place the grill pan accessory in the air fryer.
4) Put the chicken on the grill pan and cook for 40 minutes. Flip the chicken every 10 minutes to grill evenly.

5) Meanwhile, squeeze the remaining marinade in a saucepan and allow it to simmer until thickened.

6) Once cooked, brush the chicken with the sauce and garnish it with chives and lemon wedges.

Nutrition information:

- Calories per serving: 524
- Carbs: 32.4g
- Protein: 25.1g
- Fat: 32.7g

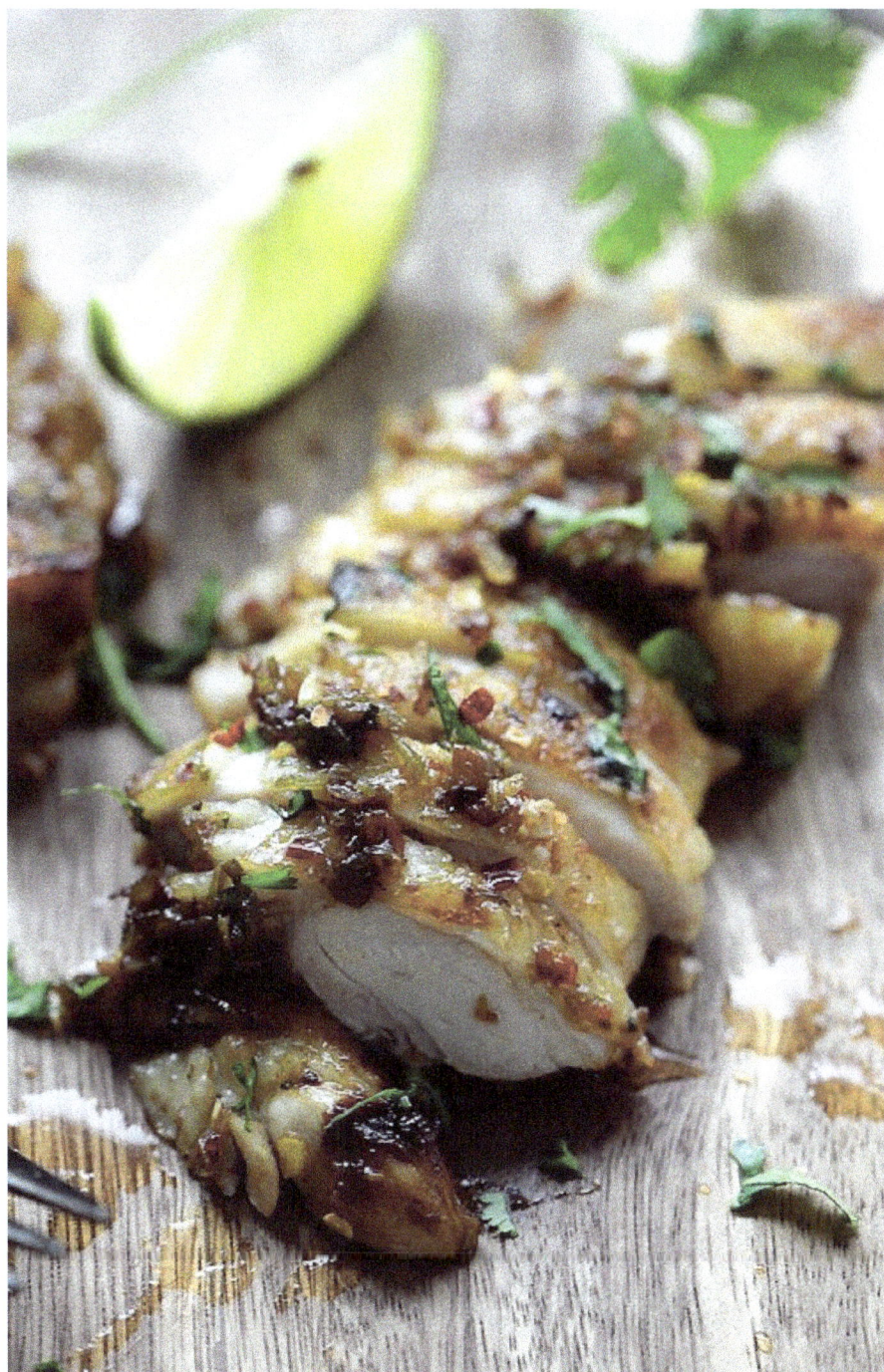

Healthy Turkey Shepherd's Pie

Servings per Recipe: 2

Cooking Time: 50 minutes

Ingredients:

- 1 tablespoon butter, room temperature /15G
- 1/2 clove garlic, minced
- 1/2 large carrot, shredded
- 1/2 onion, chopped
- 1/2 teaspoon chicken bouillon powder /2.5G
- 1/2-pound ground turkey /225G
- 1/8 teaspoon dried thyme /0.625G
- 1-1/2 large potatoes, peeled
- 1-1/2 teaspoons all-purpose flour /7.5G
- 1-1/2 teaspoons chopped fresh parsley /7.5G
- 1-1/2 teaspoons organic olive oil /7.5ML
- 2 tablespoons warm milk /30ML
- 4.5-ounce can sliced mushrooms /135G
- ground black pepper to taste
- salt to taste

Instructions:

1) Boil potatoes. Drain and transfer to a bowl. Mash with milk and butter until creamy. Set aside.

2) Grease a baking pan of air fryer with organic olive oil. Add onion and cook for 5 minutes, at 360° F or 183°C . Add chicken bouillon, garlic, thyme, parsley, mushrooms, carrot, and ground turkey. Cook for additional 10 minutes while stirring and mashing halfway through cooking time.
3) Season with pepper and salt. Stir in flour and mix well. Cook for two minutes.
4) Evenly spread turkey mixture. Top with mashed potatoes.
5) Cook for 20 minutes or until potatoes are lightly browned.
6) Serve and enjoy.

Nutrition Information:

- Calories per Serving: 342
- Carbs: 38.0g
- Protein: 18.3g
- Fat: 12.9g

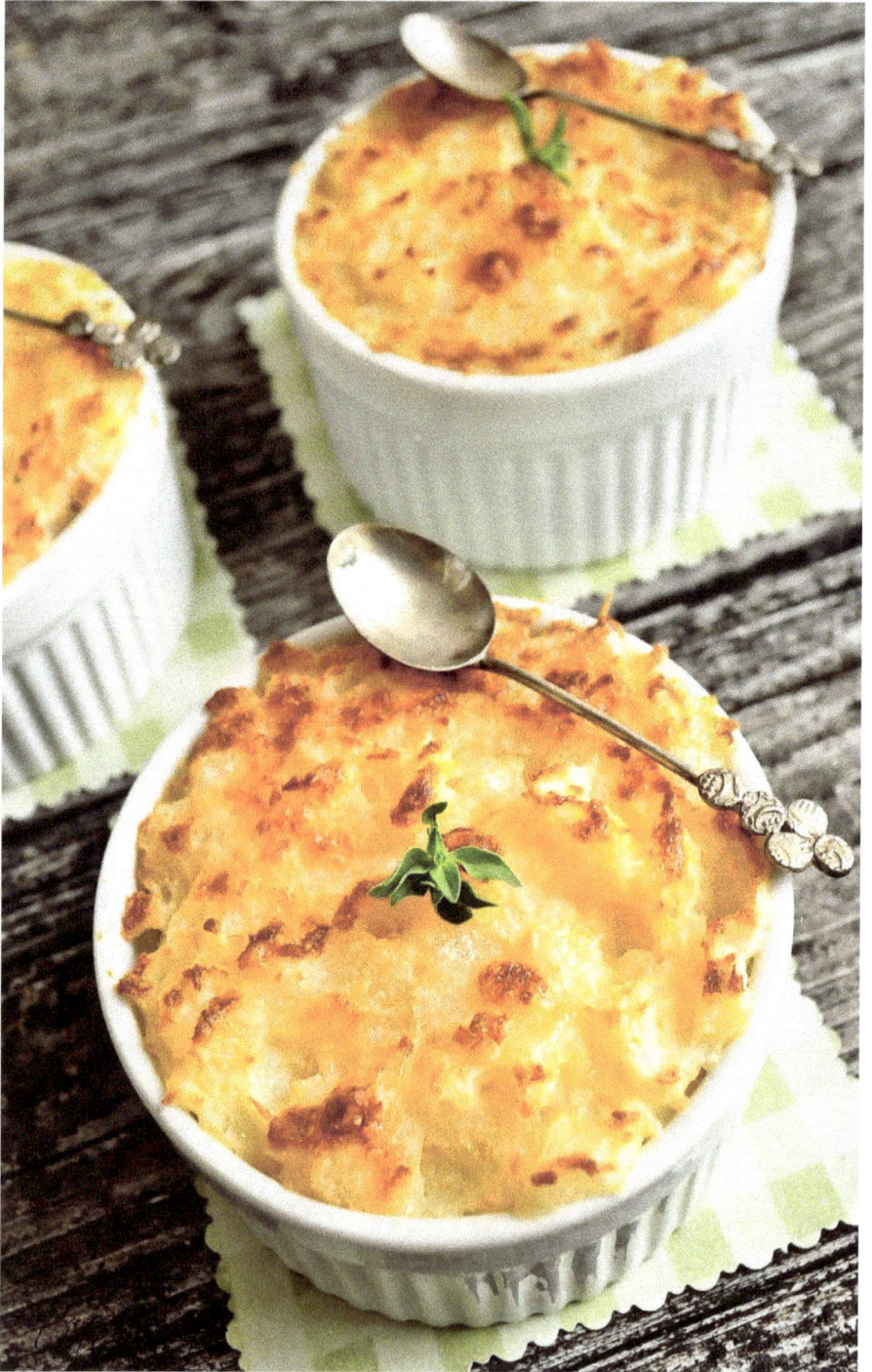

Honey & Sriracha Over Chicken

Servings per Recipe: 4

Cooking Time: 40 minutes

Ingredients:

- ½ teaspoon garlic powder /2.5G
- ½ teaspoon paprika /2.5G
- 1 tablespoon honey /15ML
- 1 teaspoon Dijon mustard /5G
- 2 tablespoons sriracha /30ML
- 3 tablespoons rice vinegar /45ML
- 4 chicken breasts
- Salt and pepper to taste

Instructions:

1) Put all ingredients in a Ziploc bag, close the zip, mix the ingredients inside the Ziploc bag. Place in a fridge for 2 hours to allow it to marinate.
2) Preheat the air fryer to 390° F or 199°C .
3) Place the grill pan accessory within the air fryer.
4) Grill the chicken for 40 minutes or more and flip the chicken every 10 minutes for even cooking.

Nutrition information:

- Calories per serving: 510

- Carbs: 6.1g
- Protein: 60.8g
- Fat: 26.9g

Honey, Lime, And Garlic Chicken BBQ

Servings per Recipe: 4

Cooking Time: 40 minutes

Ingredients

- ¼ cup lime juice, freshly squeezed /62.5ML
- ½ cup cilantro, chopped finely /32.5G
- ½ cup honey /125ML
- 1 tablespoon organic olive oil /15ML
- 2 cloves of garlic, minced
- 2 pounds boneless chicken breasts /900G
- 2 tablespoons soy sauce /30ML
- Salt and pepper to taste

Instructions:

1) Place all ingredients in the Ziploc bag and mix all ingredients to combine well. Place in a fridge for some hours.
2) Preheat the air fryer to 390° F or 199°C .
3) Place the grill pan in the air fryer.
4) Grill the chicken for 40 minutes and turn over the chicken every 10 minutes to grill evenly on every side.

Nutrition information:

- Calories per serving: 458

- Carbs: 38.9g
- Protein:52.5 g
- Fat: 10.2g

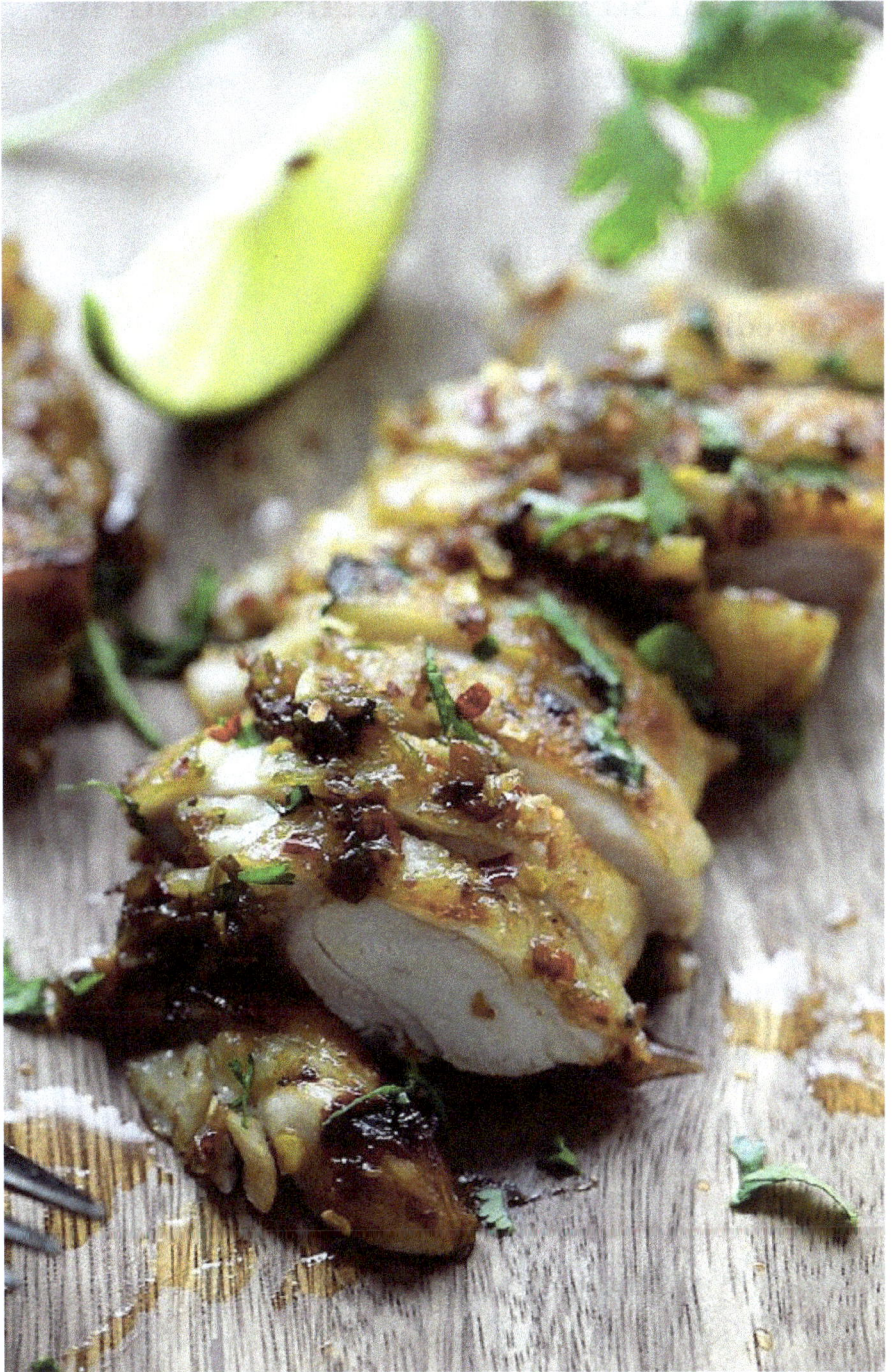

Chicken Strips with Garlic, Onion 'n Paprika Blend

Serves: 4

Cooking Time: 25 minutes

Ingredients:

- ¼ cup vegetable oil /62.5ML
- 1 cup coconut milk /250ML
- 1 tablespoon cayenne /15G
- 1 teaspoon garlic powder /5G
- 1 teaspoon onion powder /5G
- 1-pound chicken breast, cut into strips /450G
- 2 cups almond flour /260G
- 2 eggs
- 2 tablespoons paprika /30G
- Salt and pepper to taste

Instructions:

1) Place chicken meat in a bowl. Season with salt and pepper to taste. Set aside.
2) In a mixing bowl, combine the eggs and coconut milk. Set aside.
3) In another bowl, mix the almond flour, paprika, garlic powder, and onion powder.

4) Soak the chicken meat within the egg mixture then dredge within the flour mixture.

5) Place in the air fryer basket.

6) Cook for 25 minutes at 350° F or 177°C .

7) Meanwhile, prepare the new sauce by combining the red pepper cayenne and vegetable.

8) Sprinkle over chicken once cooked.

Nutrition information:

- Calories per serving: 539.7
- Carbohydrates: 8.6g
- Protein: 29.8g
- Fat: 42.9g

Chicken Tikka Masala Kebab

Servings per Recipe: 4

Cooking Time: 20 Minutes

Ingredients:

1 boneless, skinless chicken white meat, cut into bite-sized pieces

- 1 cup thick yogurt /250ML
- 1 medium bell pepper, cut into bite-sized pieces
- 1 tbsp fresh ginger paste /15G
- 1 tsp Garam masala /5G
- 1 tsp turmeric powder /5G
- 2 tbsp coriander powder /30G
- 2 tbsp cumin powder /30G
- 2 tbsp red chili powder /30G
- 2 tsp olive oil /10ML
- 8 cherry tomatoes
- Salt to taste

Instructions:

1) Add all ingredients except for chicken, bell pepper, and tomatoes in a bowl. Mix well. Add chicken, mix, place in a fridge and marinate for about an hour.

2) Skewer chicken, bell pepper, chicken, cherry tomato, chicken, then tomato and pepper. Repeat for remaining skewers.

3) Place skewer in skewer rack, for 10 minutes, cook on 390° F or 199°C . After 5 minutes turnover skewer to cook evenly.

4) Serve and enjoy.

Nutrition Information:

- Calories per Serving: 273
- Carbs: 17.4g
- Protein: 20.3g
- Fat: 13.5g

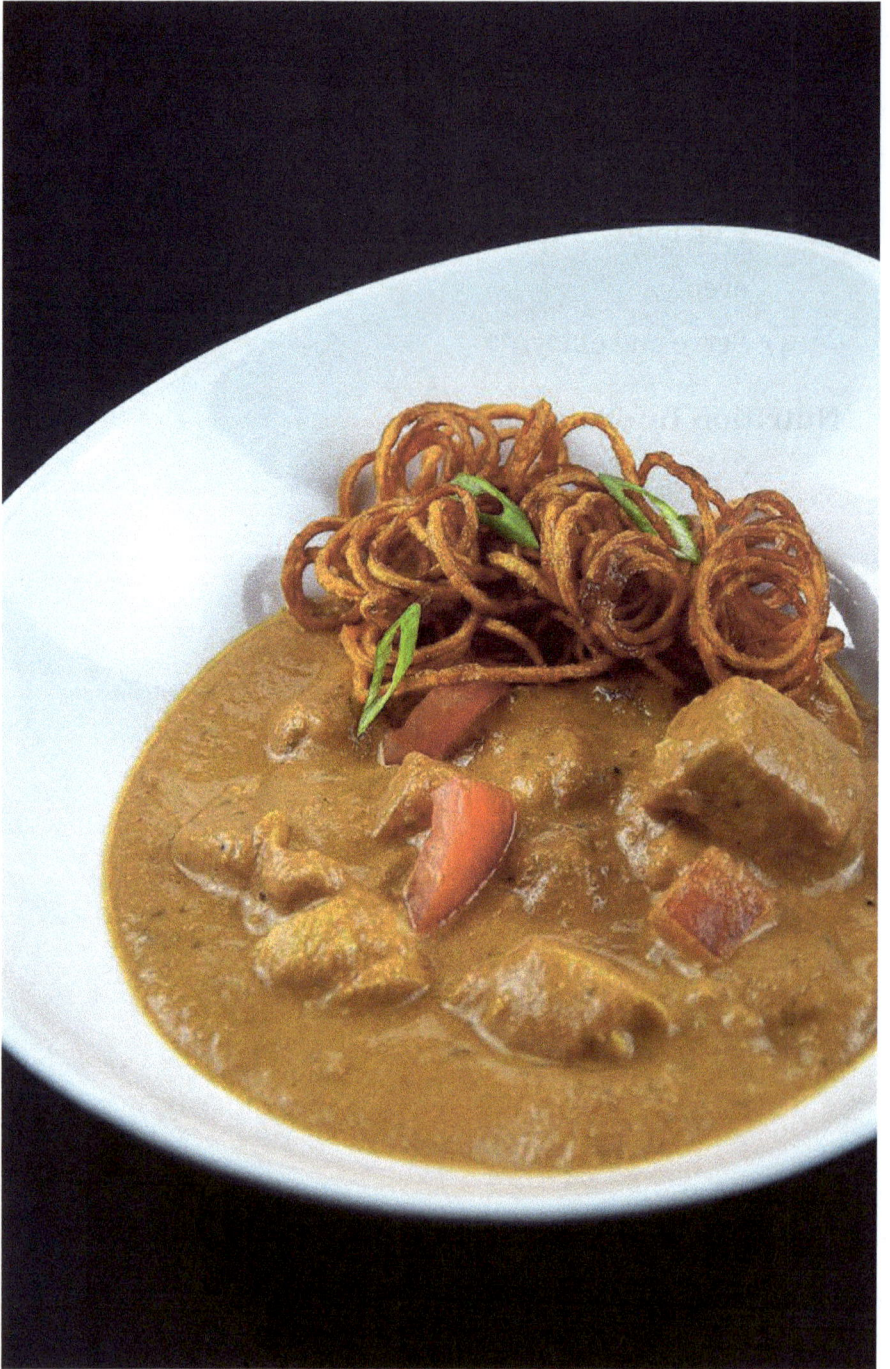

Chicken with Ginger-Cilantro Coconut Milk Marinade

Serves: 5

Cooking Time: 20 minutes

Ingredients:

- ¼ cup cilantro leaves, chopped /32.5G
- ½ cup coconut milk /125ML
- 1 tablespoon grated ginger /15G
- 1 tablespoon minced garlic /15G
- 1 teaspoon garam masala /5G
- 1 teaspoon smoked paprika /5G
- 1 teaspoon turmeric /5G
- 1-pound chicken tenders, cut by 50 per cent /450G
- Salt and pepper to taste

Instructions

1) Place all ingredients in a bowl and stir to coat the chicken tenders.
2) Allow to marinate inside the fridge for a couple of hours.
3) Preheat mid-air fryer for 5 minutes.
4) Place the chicken pieces in the air fryer basket.
5) Cook for 20 minutes at 400° F or 205°C .

Nutrition information:

- Calories per serving: 1198
- Carbohydrates: 19.5g
- Protein: 15.8g
- Fat: 117.4

Chicken with Peach Glaze

Servings per Recipe: 4

Cooking Time: 40 minutes

Ingredients:

- 1 jalapeno chopped
- 1 tablespoon chili powder /15G
- 1 tablespoon minced garlic /15G
- 1 tablespoons Dijon mustard /15G
- 2 cups peach preserves /260G
- 2 pounds chicken thighs /900G
- 2 tablespoons soy sauce /30ML
- 3 tablespoons olive oil /45ML
- Salt and pepper to taste

Instructions:

1) Place all ingredients inside a Ziploc bag and allow to set in the fridge for 2 hours.
2) Preheat the air fryer to 390° F or 199°C .
3) Place the grill pan accessory in the air fryer.
4) Grill for 40 minutes while turning over the chicken every 10 minutes.
5) Meanwhile, pour the marinade in a saucepan and allow to simmer for 5 minutes until the sauce thickens.
6) Brush the chicken with the sauce before serving.

Nutrition information:

- Calories per serving: 730
- Carbs: 31.7g
- Protein: 39.4g
- Fat: 49.5g

Chicken-Parm, Broccoli 'n Mushroom Bake

Servings per Recipe: 2

Cooking Time: 40 minutes

Ingredients:

- 1 (13.5 ounces) can spinach, drained /405G
- 1 cup shredded mozzarella cheese /130G
- 1/2 (10.75 ounces) can condensed cream of mushroom soup /322.5ML
- 1/3 cup bacon bits /43G
- 1/4 cup grated Parmesan cheese /32.5G
- 1/4 cup half-and-half /32.5G
- 1-1/2 teaspoons Italian seasoning /7.5G
- 1-1/2 teaspoons freshly squeezed lemon juice /7.5ML
- 1-1/2 teaspoons minced garlic /7.5ML
- 2 ounces fresh mushrooms, sliced /60G
- 2 skinless, boneless chicken halves
- 2 tablespoons butter /30G

Instructions:

1) Lightly grease the baking pan. Add chicken breast, cook for 20 minutes at 360° F or 183°C . Turnover the chicken breast after 10 minutes of cooking. After which you can transfer it to a plate and set it aside.

2) In the same baking pan, melt butter. Stir in Parmesan cheese, half and half, Italian seasoning, mushroom soup, fresh lemon juice, and garlic. Mix well and cook for 5 minutes or until well cooked.

3) Stir in spinach and chicken. Top with bacon bits and mozzarella cheese.

4) Cook for 15 minutes at 390° F or 199°C until tops are lightly browned.

5) Serve and enjoy.

Nutrition Information:

- Calories per Serving: 659
- Carbs: 17.6g
- Protein: 61.6g
- Fat: 38.0g

Simple Herbs de Provence Pork Loin Roast

Servings per Recipe: 4

Cooking Time: 35 minutes

Ingredients:

- 4 pounds pork loin /1800G
- A pinch of garlic salt
- A pinch of herbs de Provence

Instructions:

1) Preheat the air fryer to 330° F or 166°C .
2) Season pork using garlic salt and herbs,
3) Place in the air fryer grill pan.
4) Cook for 30 to 35 minutes.

Nutrition information:

- Calories per serving: 922
- Carbs: 0.9g
- Protein: 116.7g
- Fat: 50.2g

Simple Lamb BBQ with Herbed Salt

Servings per Recipe: 8

Cooking Time: one hour 20 Minutes

Ingredients:

- 2 ½ tablespoons herb salt /37.5G
- 2 tablespoons extra virgin olive oil /30ML
- 4 pounds boneless leg of lamb, cut into 2-inch chunks /1800G

Instructions:

1) Preheat air fryer to 390° F or 199°C .
2) Place the grill pan accessory in the air fryer.
3) Season the meat while using herb salt and brush with extra virgin olive oil.
4) Grill the meat for 20 minutes per batch.
5) Make sure to turn over the meat every 10 minutes for cooking.

Nutrition information:

- Calories per serving: 347
- Carbs: 0g
- Protein: 46.6g
- Fat: 17.8g

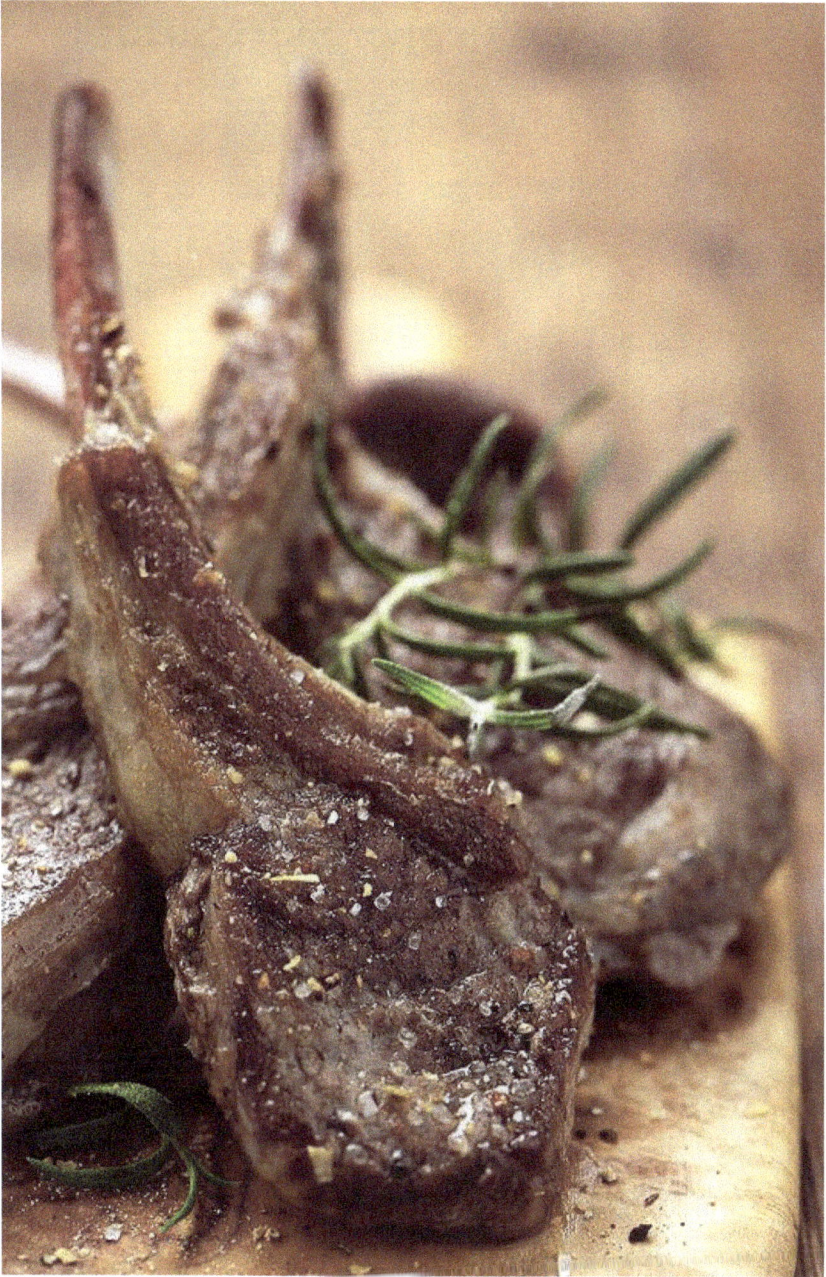

Simple Salt and Pepper Skirt Steak

Servings per Recipe: 3

Cooking Time: 30 minutes

Ingredients:

- 1 ½ pounds skirt steak /675G
- Salt and pepper to taste

Instructions:

1) Preheat mid-air fryer to 390° F or 199°C .
2) Place the grill pan accessory in the mid-air fryer.
3) Season the skirt steak with salt and pepper to taste.
4) Place the grill pan and cook for 15 minutes per batch.
5) Flip the meat halfway through the cooking time.

Nutrition information:

- Calories per serving: 469
- Carbs: 1g
- Protein: 60g
- Fat: 25g

Sirloin with Yogurt 'n Curry-Paprika

Servings per Recipe: 3

Cooking Time: 25 minutes

Ingredients:

- ¼ cup mint, chopped /32.5G
- ½ cup low-fat yogurt /125ML
- 1 ½ pounds boneless beef top loin steak /675G
- 2 teaspoons curry powder /10G
- 2 teaspoons paprika /10G
- 3 tablespoons freshly squeezed lemon juice /45ML
- 6 cloves of garlic, minced
- Salt and pepper to taste

Instructions:

1) Place all ingredients except the green onions in a Ziploc bag and allow to marinate inside the fridge for around 120 minutes.
2) Preheat the air fryer to 390° F or 199°C .
3) Place the grill pan accessory in the mid-air fryer.
4) Grill for 25 minutes to a half-hour.
5) Flip the steaks regularly until completely grilled.

Nutrition information:

- Calories per serving: 596

- Carbs: 8.9g
- Protein: 70.5g
- Fat: 30.9g

Skirt Steak BBQ Recipe from Korea

Servings per Recipe: 1

Cooking Time: 30 Minutes

Ingredients

- 1 skirt steak, halved
- 3 tablespoons gochujang sauce /45ML
- 3 tablespoons olive oil /45ML
- 3 tablespoons rice vinegar /45ML
- Salt and pepper to taste

Instructions:

1) Preheat the air fryer to 390° F or 199°C .
2) Place the grill pan accessory in the air fryer.
3) Rub all spices and seasonings on the skirt steak.
4) Place on the grill and cook for 15 minutes per batch.
5) Flip the steak after 7 **1/2** minutes of cooking time.
6) Serve with gochujang or kimchi.

Nutrition information:

- Calories per serving: 467
- Carbs: 8.3g
- Protein:9.3 g
- Fat: 44g

Hanger Steak in Mole Rub

Servings per Recipe: 2

Cooking Time: an hour

Ingredients:

- 1 tablespoon ground black pepper /15G
- 2 hanger steaks
- 2 tablespoons coriander seeds /30G
- 2 tablespoons ground coffee /30G
- 2 tablespoons olive oil /30ML
- 2 tablespoons salt /30G
- 4 teaspoons unsweetened powdered cocoa /20G
- 4 teaspoons brown sugar /20G

Instructions:

1) Preheat the air fryer to 390° F or 199°C .
2) Place the grill pan in the air fryer.
3) Combine the coriander seeds, ground coffee, salt, brown sugar, hot chocolate mix, and black pepper in a bowl and mix well.
4) Rub the spice mixture lavishly on the steaks and brush with oil.
5) Grill for 30 Minutes and ensure to turn over the meat every 10 minutes after only grilling and cook in batches.

Nutrition information:

- Calories per serving: 680

- Carbs: 16g
- Protein:48 g
- Fat: 47g

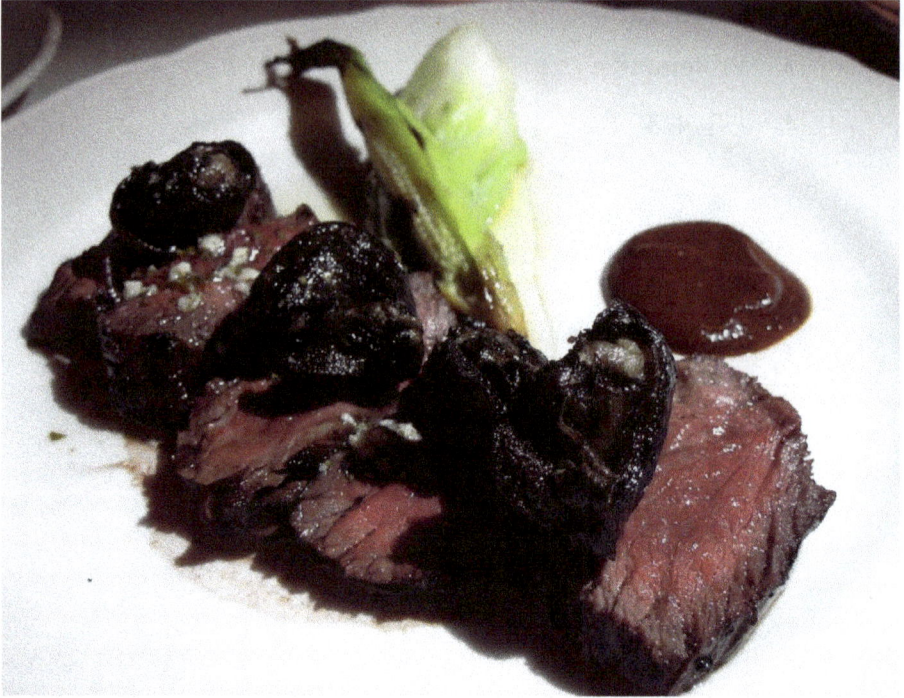

Hickory Smoked Beef Jerky

Servings per Recipe: 2

Cooking Time: an hour

Ingredients:

- ¼ cup Worcestershire sauce /62.5ML
- ½ cup brown sugar /65G
- ½ cup soy sauce /125ML
- ½ teaspoon black pepper /2.5G
- ½ teaspoon smoked paprika /2.5G
- 1 tablespoon chili pepper sauce /15ML
- 1 tablespoon liquid smoke, hickory /15ML
- 1 teaspoon garlic powder /5G
- 1 teaspoon onion powder /5G
- 1-pound ground beef, sliced thinly /450G

Instructions:

1) Add all ingredients inside a mixing bowl or Ziploc bag.
2) Marinate in the fridge overnight.
3) Preheat air fryer to 330° F or 166°C .
4) Place the beef slices on the double layer rack.
5) Cook for an hour until beef is dry.

Nutrition information:

- Calories per serving: 723
- Carbs: 79.8g

- Protein: 55.6g
- Fat: 20.2g

Italian Beef Roast

Serves: 10

Cooking Time: 3 hours

Ingredients:

- ¼ teaspoon black pepper /1.25G
- ½ cup water /125ML
- ½ teaspoon thyme /2.5G
- 1 onion, sliced thinly
- 1 teaspoon basil /5G
- 1 teaspoon salt /5G
- 2 ½ pounds beef round roast /1125G
- 4 tablespoons extra virgin olive oil /60ML

Instructions:

1) Place all ingredients in the baking dish so that it covers the surface of the dish.
2) Place the baking dish in the air fryer. Close.
3) Cook for 3 hours at 400° F or 205°C .

Nutrition information:

- Calories per serving: 282
- Carbohydrates: 0.2g
- Protein: 23.6g
- Fat: 20.7g

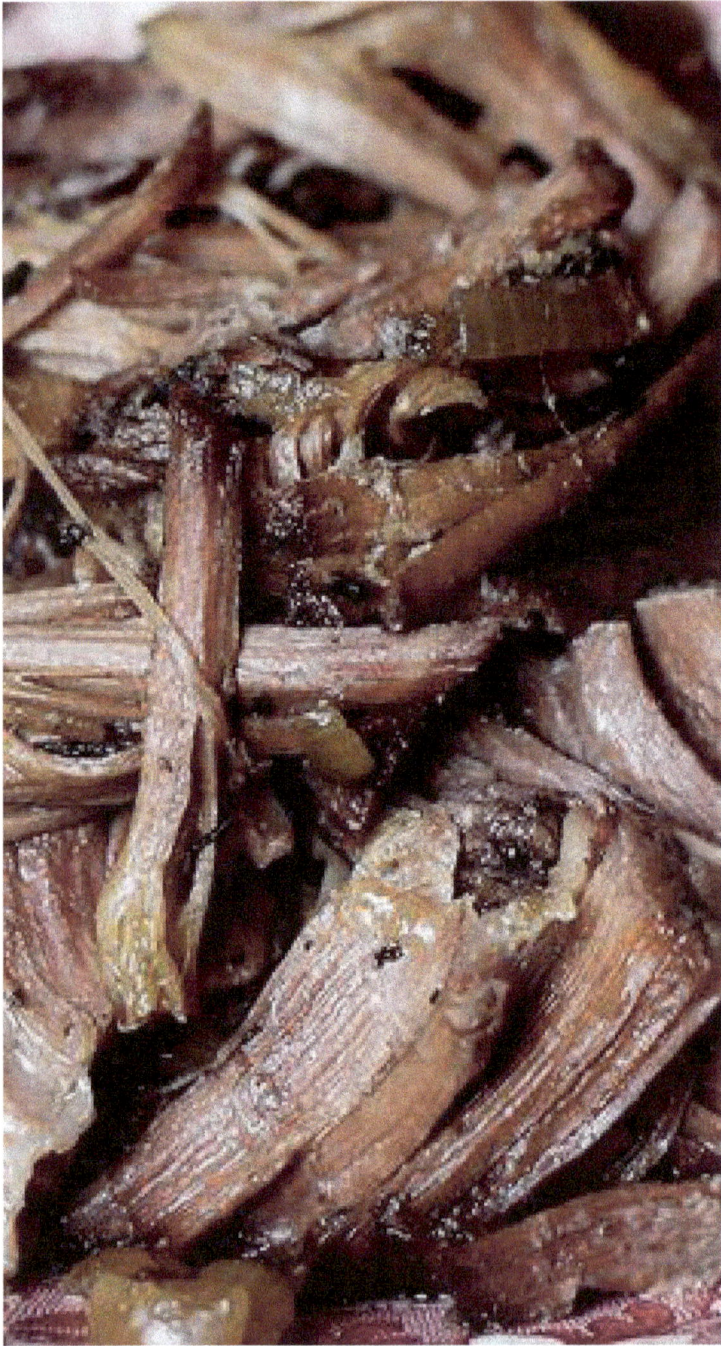

Italian Sausage & Tomato Egg Bake

Servings per Recipe: 1

Cooking Time: 16 minutes

Ingredients:

- ½ Italian sausage, sliced into ¼-inch thick
- 1 tablespoon extra-virgin olive oil /15ML
- 3 eggs
- 4 cherry tomatoes (by 50 %)
- Chopped parsley
- Grano Padano cheese (or parmesan)
- Salt/Pepper

Instructions:

1) Grease baking pan of air fryer lightly with cooking spray.
2) Add Italian sausage and cook for 5 minutes at 360° F or 183°C .
3) Add extra virgin olive oil and cherry tomatoes. Cook for an additional 6 minutes.
4) Meanwhile, whisk eggs, parsley, cheese, salt, and pepper well in the bowl.
5) Remove the basket and chuck the ball mixture slightly. Pour eggs over the mixture.
6) Cook for an additional 5 minutes.
7) Serve and enjoy.

Nutrition Information:

- Calories per Serving: 295
- Carbs: 7.8g
- Protein: 14.4g
- Fat: 22.9g

Keto-Approved Cheeseburger Bake

Servings per Recipe: 4

Cooking Time: 35 minutes

Ingredients:

- 1 clove garlic, minced
- 1/2 cup heavy whipping cream /125ML
- 1/2-pound bacon, cut into small pieces /225G
- 1/4 teaspoon onion powder /1.25G
- 1/4 teaspoon salt /1.25G
- 1/8 teaspoon ground black pepper /0.625G
- 1-pound ground beef /450G
- 4 eggs
- 6-ounce shredded Cheddar cheese, divided /180G

Instructions:

1) Grease baking pan of air fryer lightly with cooking spray. Add beef, onion powder, and garlic. For 10 Minutes, cook at 360° **OR** 183°C . Stir and crush every 5 minutes.

2) Remove excess fat and evenly spread ground beef in the pan. Evenly spread bacon slices on the top. Sprinkle 50% of the cheese ahead.

3) Whisk well pepper, salt, heavy cream, and eggs. Pour over bacon.

4) Sprinkle the remaining cheese and then eggs.

5) Cover the pan with foil and cook for 15 minutes.

6) Remove the foil and cook for the next 10 minutes until the tops are browned and eggs are set.

7) Serve and enjoy.

Nutrition Information:

- Calories per Serving: 454
- Carbs: 1.6g
- Protein: 28.7g
- Fat: 36.9g

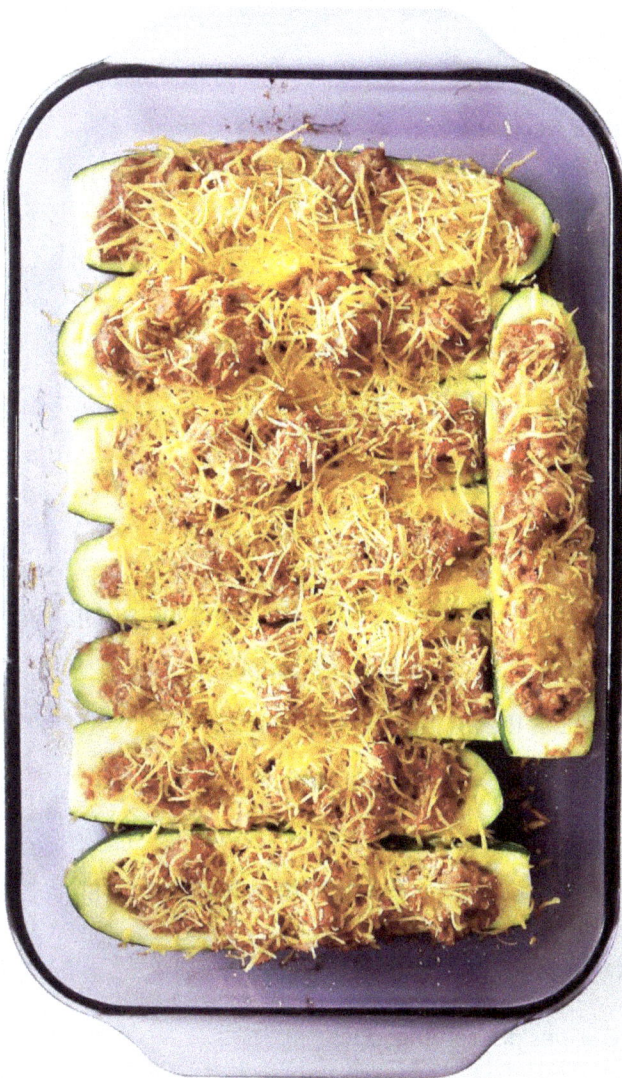

Beefy Steak Topped with Chimichurri Sauce

Servings per Recipe: 6

Cooking Time: an hour

Ingredients:

- 1 cup commercial chimichurri /250ML
- 3 pounds steak /1350G
- Salt and pepper to taste

Instructions:

1) Get a Ziploc bag and add all the ingredients to it. Place in a fridge and allow to marinate for a couple of hours.
2) Preheat the air fryer to 390° F or 199°C .
3) Place the grill pan in the air fryer.
4) Grill the skirt steak for 20 minutes per batch.
5) Flip over the steak every 10 minutes for even grilling.

Nutrition information:

- Calories per serving: 507
- Carbs: 2.8g
- Protein: 63g
- Fat: 27g

Bourbon-BBQ Sauce Marinated Beef BBQ

Servings per Recipe: 4

Cooking Time: 60 minutes

Ingredients:

- ¼ cup bourbon /62.5ML
- ¼ cup barbecue sauce /62.5ML
- 1 tablespoon Worcestershire sauce /15ML
- 2 pounds beef steak, pounded /900G
- Salt and pepper to taste

Instructions:

1) Place all ingredients in the Ziploc bag, place them in a fridge for a couple of hours to allow the ingredients to marinate.
2) Preheat the air fryer to 390 ° F or 199°C .
3) Place the grill pan accessory in the air fryer.
4) Place around the grill pan and cook for 20 minutes per batch.
5) Turnover and stir halfway the cooking time for even cooking.
6) Meanwhile, pour the marinade on the saucepan and allow it to simmer for 10 minutes
7) Serve beef with bourbon sauce.

Nutrition information:

- Calories per serving: 346

- Carbs: 9.8g
- Protein: 48.2g
- Fat: 12.6g

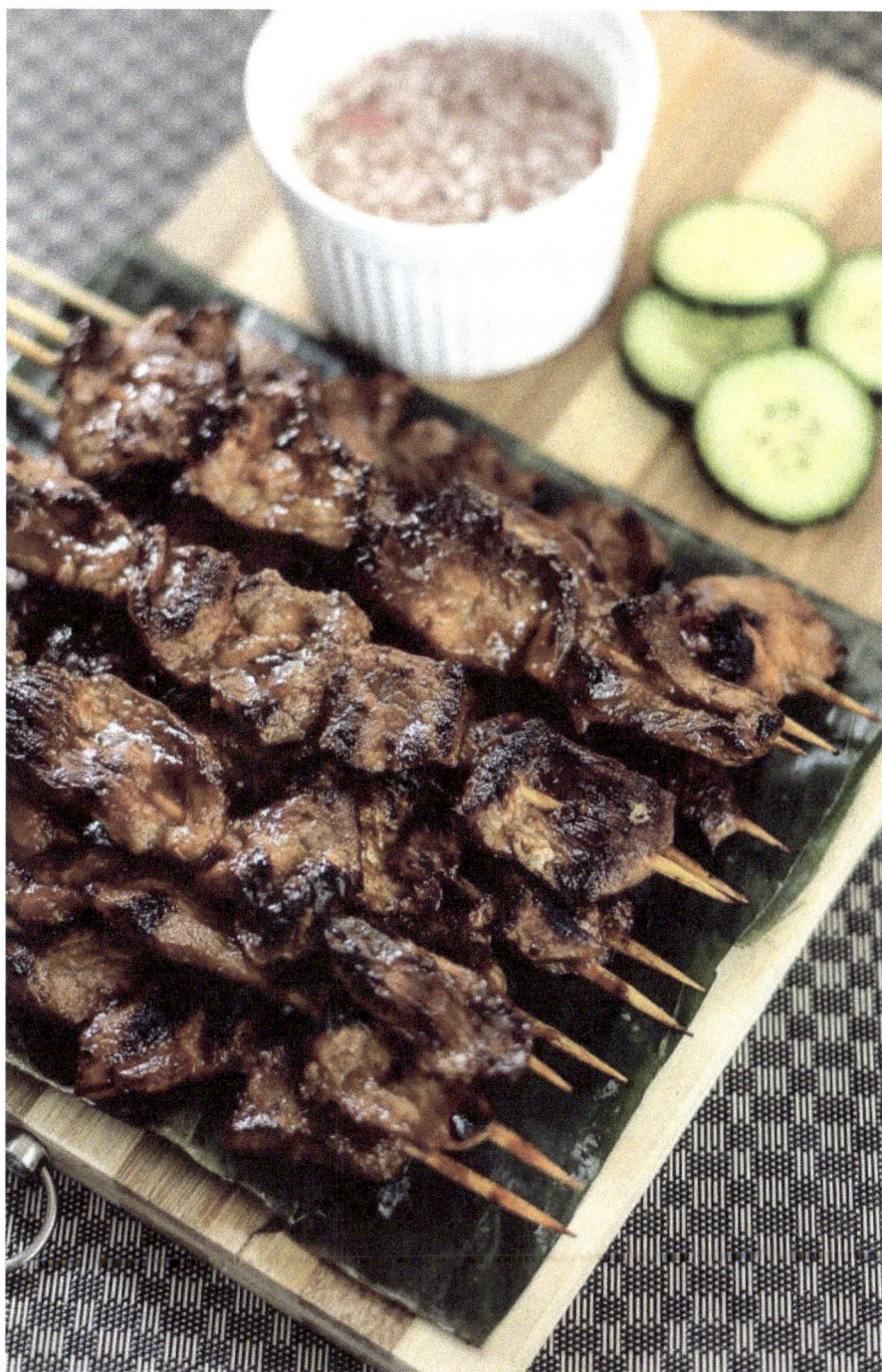

Buttered Garlic-Thyme Roast Beef

Serves: 12

Cooking Time: 2 hours

Ingredients:

- 1 ½ tablespoon garlic /22.5G
- 1 cup beef stock /250ML
- 1 teaspoon black pepper /5G
- 1 teaspoon salt /5G
- 1 teaspoon thyme leaves, chopped /5G
- 3 tablespoons butter /45G
- 3-pound eye of round roast /1350G
- 6 tablespoons organic olive oil /90ML

Instructions:

1) Get all the ingredients and add them to a Ziploc bag, place them in the fridge and allow them to marinate for a couple of hours.
2) Preheat the air fryer for 5 minutes.
3) Transfer all ingredients inside a baking dish that will fit in the air fryer.
4) Place in the air fryer and cook for a couple of hours at 400° F or 205°C .
5) Baste the beef with the sauce every 30 Minutes.

Nutrition information:

- Calories per serving: 273
- Carbohydrates: 0.8g
- Protein: 34.2g
- Fat: 14.7g

Cajun 'n Coriander Seasoned Ribs

Servings per Recipe: 4

Cooking Time: 1 hour

Ingredients:

- ¼ cup brown sugar /32.5G
- ½ teaspoon lemon /2.5G
- 1 tablespoon paprika /15G
- 1 tablespoon salt /15G
- 1 teaspoon coriander seed powder /5G
- 2 slabs spareribs
- 2 tablespoons onion powder /30G
- 2 teaspoon Cajun seasoning /10G

Instructions:

1) Preheat mid-air fryer to 390° F or 199°C .
2) Place the grill pan in the air fryer.
3) In a small bowl, combine the spices.
4) Rub the spice mixture lavishly on to the spareribs.
5) Place the spareribs around the grill pan and cook for 20 minutes per batch.
6) Serve along with your favorite barbecue sauce.

Nutrition information:

- Calories per serving: 490

- Carbs: 18.2g
- Protein: 24.4g
- Fat: 35.5g

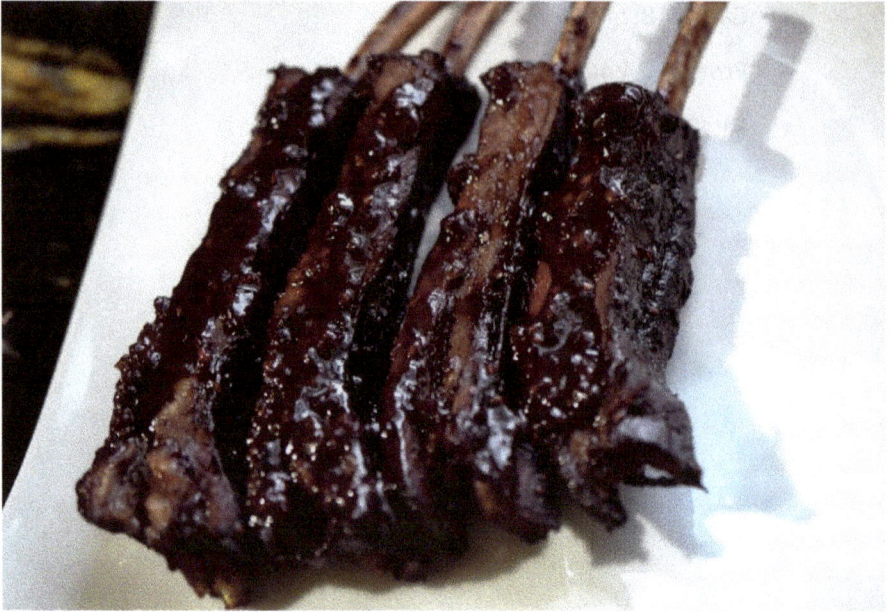

Cajun Sweet-Sour Grilled Pork

Servings per Recipe: 3

Cooking Time: 12 minutes

Ingredients:

- ¼ cup brown sugar /32.5G
- 1/4 cup cider vinegar /62.5G
- 1-lb pork loin, sliced into 1-inch cubes /450G
- 2 tablespoons Cajun seasoning /30G
- 3 tablespoons brown sugar /45G

Instructions:

1) Mix the pork loin, 3 tablespoons brown sugar, and Cajun seasoning in a shallow bowl. Mix well to coat. Marinate in the refrigerator for 3 hours.
2) Mix brown sugar and vinegar in a shallow bowl for basting.
3) Thread pork pieces in skewers. Baste with sauce and place on a skewer rack in the air fryer.
4) Cook at 360° F or 183°C for 12 minutes, turn skewer halfway through cooking time and baste with sauce. If necessary, cook in batches.
5) Serve and enjoy

Nutrition Information:

- Calories per Serving: 428

- Carbs: 30.3g
- Protein: 39.0g
- Fat: 16.7g

Crisped Baked Cheese Stuffed Chile Pepper

Servings per Recipe: 3

Cooking Time: 30 Minutes

Ingredients:

- 1 (7 ounces or 210G) can whole green Chile peppers, drained
- 1 egg, beaten
- 1 tablespoon all-purpose flour /15G
- 1/2 (5 ounces or 150ML) can evaporated milk
- 1/2 (large) can tomato sauce
- 1/4-pound Monterey Jack cheese, shredded /112.5G
- 1/4-pound Longhorn or Cheddar cheese, shredded /112.5G
- 1/4 cup milk /62.5ML

Instructions:

1) Grease baking pan, evenly spread chilies on the pan, sprinkle cheddar and Jack cheese on the top.
2) Whisk flour, milk, and eggs in a bowl and pour over chilies.
3) Cook for 20 minutes at 360° F or 183°C .
4) Add tomato sauce on top.

5) Cook for 10 minutes at 390° F or 199°C or until the tops are lightly brown.

6) Dish out and enjoy.

Nutrition Information:

- Calories per Serving: 392
- Carbs: 12.0g
- Protein: 23.9g
- Fat: 27.6g

Crisped Noodle Salad Chinese Style

Serves: 2

Cooking Time: 20 minutes

Ingredients:

- 1 carrot, sliced thinly
- 1 cup cabbage, sliced thinly /130G
- 1 green bell pepper, sliced thinly
- 1 onion, sliced thinly
- 1 package wheat noodles
- 1 sprig coriander, chopped
- 1 tablespoon olive oil /15ML
- 1 tablespoon lime juice /15ML
- 1 tablespoon red chili sauce /15ML
- 1 tablespoon tamari /15G
- 1 tomato, chopped
- salt to taste

Instructions:

1) Add a teaspoon of salt into a large pot containing water, allow to boil, add the noodles, boil until almost done. Drain with a sieve.
2) Coat noodles evenly with oil.
3) lay the air fryer basket with a thin foil and put the coated noodles inside.

4) Meanwhile, preheat the air fryer to 395° F or 202°C . Place the basket in the air fryer for 15 to 20 minutes or cook until crisp. Place in a bowl.

5) In the meantime, add the tamari, red chili sauce, and lime juice to a bowl and mix well. Season with salt and pepper to taste.

6) Add the vegetables and pour sauce over the mid air-fried noodles.

Nutrition information:

- Calories per serving: 165
- Carbohydrates: 20.41g
- Protein:4.12 g
- Fat:7.39 g

Crisped Tofu with Paprika

Serves: 4

Ingredients:

- ¼ cup cornstarch /32.5G
- 1 block extra firm tofu, pressed to remove excess water and cut into cubes
- 1 tablespoon smoked paprika /15G
- salt and pepper to taste

Instructions:

1) Line air fryer basket with aluminium foil and brush with oil.
2) Preheat air fryer to 370° F or 188°C .
3) Mix all ingredients in the bowl. Toss to blend.
4) Place in the air fryer basket and cook for 12 minutes.

Nutrition information:

- Calories per serving: 155
- Carbohydrates:11.56 g
- Protein:11.74 g
- Fat:6.88 g

Crispy 'n Healthy Avocado Fingers

Serves: 4

Cooking Time: 10 Minutes

Ingredients:

- ½ cup panko breadcrumbs /65G
- ½ teaspoon salt /2.5G
- 1 pitted Haas avocado, peeled and sliced
- liquid from 1 can of white beans or aquafaba

Instructions:

1) Preheat mid-air fryer at 350° F or 177°C .
2) Mix the breadcrumbs and salt in a bowl until well combined.
3) Dip the avocado slices inside the aquafaba and then in the breadcrumb mixture.
4) Place the avocado slices one after the other in a single layer in the air fryer basket.
5) Cook for 10 minutes and shake frequently for even doneness.

Nutrition information:

- Calories per serving: 51
- Carbohydrates: 6.45g
- Protein: 1.39g

- Fat: 7.51g

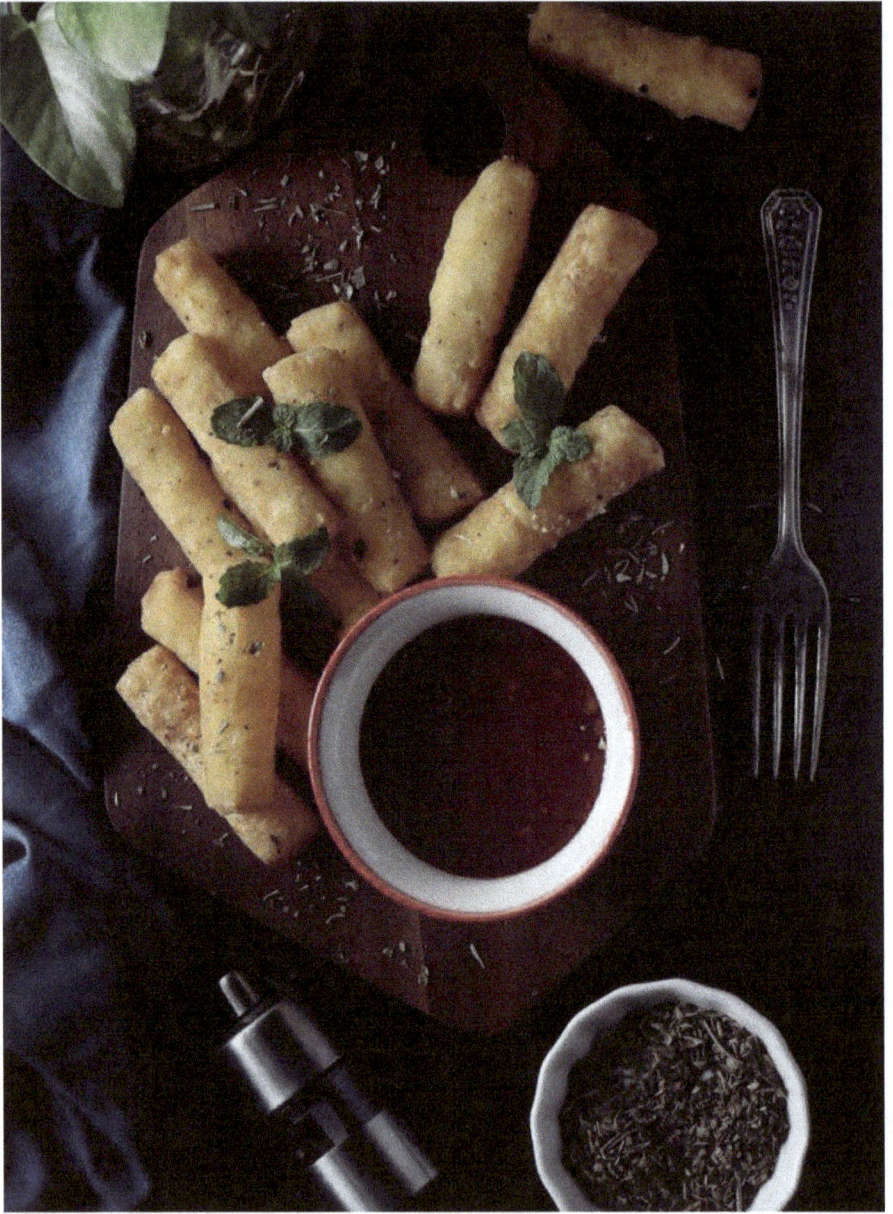

Crispy 'n Savory Spring Rolls

Serves: 4

Cooking Time: 15

Ingredients:

- ½ teaspoon ginger, finely chopped /2.5G
- 1 celery stalk, chopped
- 1 cup shiitake mushroom, sliced thinly /65G
- 1 medium carrot, shredded
- 1 tablespoon soy sauce /15ML
- 1 teaspoon coconut sugar /5G
- 1 teaspoon corn starch + 2 tablespoon water /5G + 30ML
- 1 teaspoon nutritional yeast /5G
- 8 spring roll wrappers

Instructions:

1) Mix the celery stalk, carrots, ginger, coconut sugar, soy sauce and nutritional yeast properly.
2) Place a tablespoon of vegetable oil in the middle of the spring roll wrappers.
3) Roll and seal the edges of the wrapper using the cornstarch mixture.
4) Cook in a preheated air fryer to 400° F or 205°C for 15 or until the spring roll wrapper is crispy.

Nutrition information:

- Calories per serving: 118
- Carbohydrates: 15g
- Protein: 10g
- Fat: 2g

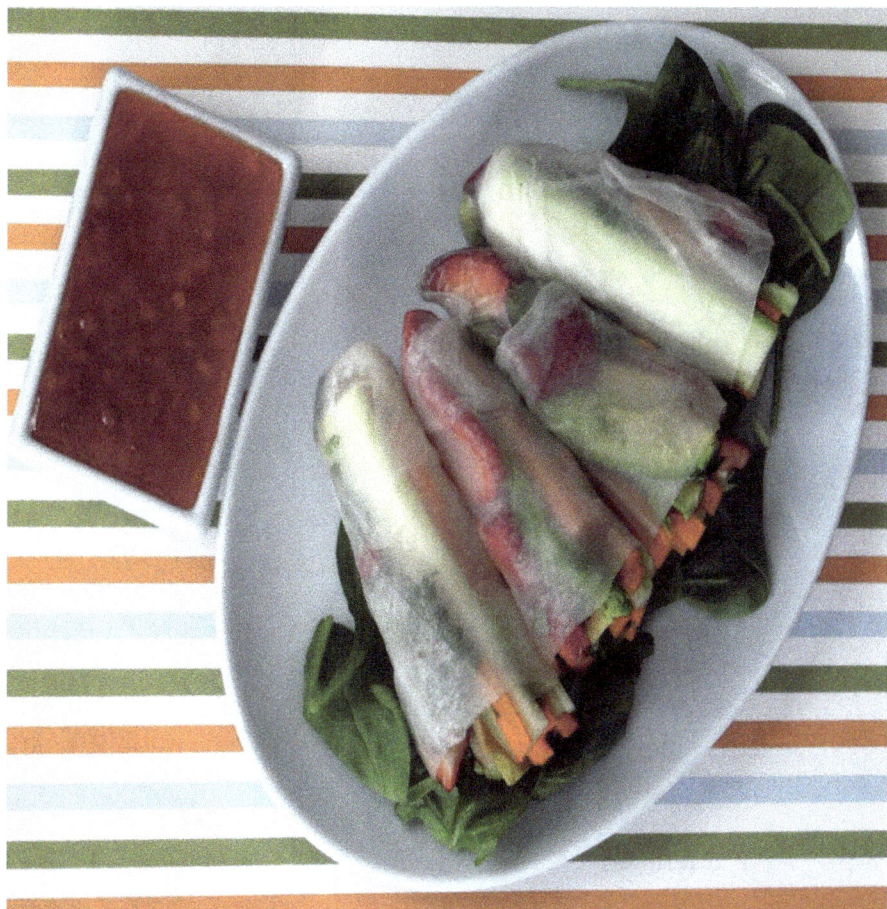

Buttered Baked Cod with Wine

Servings per Recipe: 2

Cooking Time: 12 minutes

Ingredients:

- 1 tablespoon butter /15g
- 1 tablespoon butter /15g
- 2 tablespoons dry white wine /30g
- 1/2 pound thick-cut cod loin /225g
- 1-1/2 teaspoons chopped fresh parsley /7.5g
- 1-1/2 teaspoons chopped green onion /7.5g
- 1/2 lemon, cut into wedges
- 1/4 sleeve buttery round crackers (for example Ritz®), crushed
- 1/4 lemon, juiced

Instructions

1) Put butter in a bowl, place in a microwave to melt and whisk in the crackers.
2) Lightly brush some butter in the baking pan. Place the baking pan in the air fryer and heat for two minutes at 3900 F or 199°C.
3) Grab a small bowl, mix lemon juice, white wine, parsley, and green onion. Whisk well to combine.

4) Dip the cod filets in melted butter. Pour the dressing on it. Add the butter-cracker mixture.

5) Cook for 10 Minutes at 3900 F or 199°C in the air fryer.

6) Serve with a dashing slice of lemon juice.

Nutrition Information:

- Calories per Serving: 266
- Carbs: 9.3g
- Protein: 20.9g
- Fat: 16.1g

Buttered Garlic-Oregano on Clams

Servings per Recipe: 4

Cooking Time: 5 minutes

Ingredients:

- ¼ cup mozzarella, grated /32.5g
- ¼ cup parsley, chopped /32.5g
- 1 cup breadcrumbs /130g
- 1 teaspoon dried oregano /5g
- 2 dozen clams, shucked
- 3 cloves of garlic, minced
- 4 tablespoons butter, melted /60ml

Instructions:

1) While preheating your air fryer to 3900 F or 199°C add the breadcrumbs, parmesan cheese, parsley, oregano, and garlic in a medium-size bowl and stir in the melted butter.
2) Fill the baking pan with the clams.
3) Sprinkle the crumb mixture on the clams and place it in the air fryer.
4) Cook for 5 minutes.

Nutrition information:

- Calories per serving: 160

- Carbs: 6.3g
- Protein: 2.9g
- Fat: 13.6g

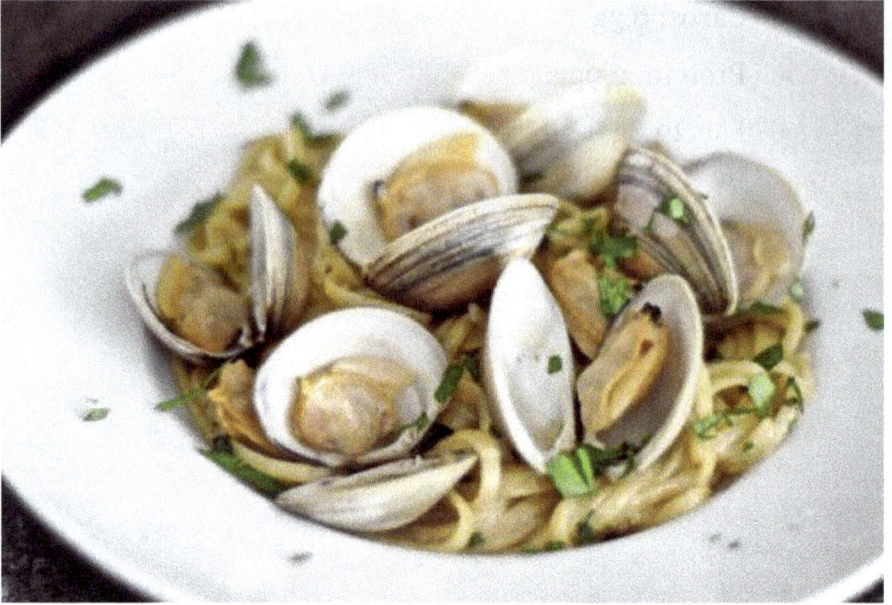

Butterflied Prawns with Garlic-Sriracha

Servings per Recipe: 2

Cooking Time: 15

Ingredients:

- 1 tablespoon lime juice /15ml
- 1 tablespoon sriracha /15g
- 1-pound large prawns, shells removed and cut lengthwise or butterflied /450g
- 1 teaspoon fish sauce /5ml
- 2 tablespoons melted butter /30ml
- 2 tablespoons minced garlic /30g
- Salt and pepper to taste

Instructions:

1) Preheat the air fryer to 3900 F or 199°C using the air fryer setting.
2) Place the grill pan in the mid-air fryer.
3) Spice the prawns with all other mentioned ingredients.
4) Place in the grill pan and cook for 15 minutes. Flip over halfway through cooking time.

Nutrition information:

- Calories per serving: 443
- Carbs:9.7 g

- Protein: 62.8g
- Fat: 16.9g

Cajun Seasoned Salmon Filet

Serves: 1

Cooking Time: 15

Ingredients:

- 1 salmon fillet
- 1 teaspoon juice from lemon, freshly squeezed /5ml
- 3 tablespoons extra virgin essential olive oil /45ml
- A dash of Cajun seasoning mix
- Salt and pepper to taste

Instructions:

1) Preheat the air fryer for 5 minutes using the air fryer setting.
2) Place all ingredients inside a bowl, mix well to coat.
3) Place the fish fillet in the air fryer's basket.
4) Bake for 15 minutes at 3250 F or 163°C .
5) Once cooked brush with extra virgin olive oil

Nutrition information:

- Calories per serving: 523
- Carbohydrates: 4.6g
- Protein: 47.9g
- Fat: 34.8g

Cajun Spiced Lemon-Shrimp Kebabs

Servings per Recipe: 2

Cooking Time: 10 minutes

Ingredients:

- 1 tsp cayenne /5g
- 1 tsp garlic powder /5g
- 1 tsp kosher salt /5g
- 1 tsp onion powder /5g
- 1 tsp oregano /5g
- 1 tsp paprika /5g
- 12 pcs XL shrimp
- 2 lemons, sliced thinly crosswise
- 2 tbsp extra virgin olive oil /30ml

Instructions:

1) Mix all ingredients except the lemons. Marinate for 10 minutes.
2) Fasten 3 shrimps on a steel skewer.
3) Place the above in a skewer rack.
4) Cook for 5 minutes at 3900 F or 199°C .
5) Squeeze lemon juice on the shrimps and serve.

Nutrition Information:

- Calories per Serving: 232

- Carbs: 7.9g
- Protein: 15.9g
- Fat: 15.1g

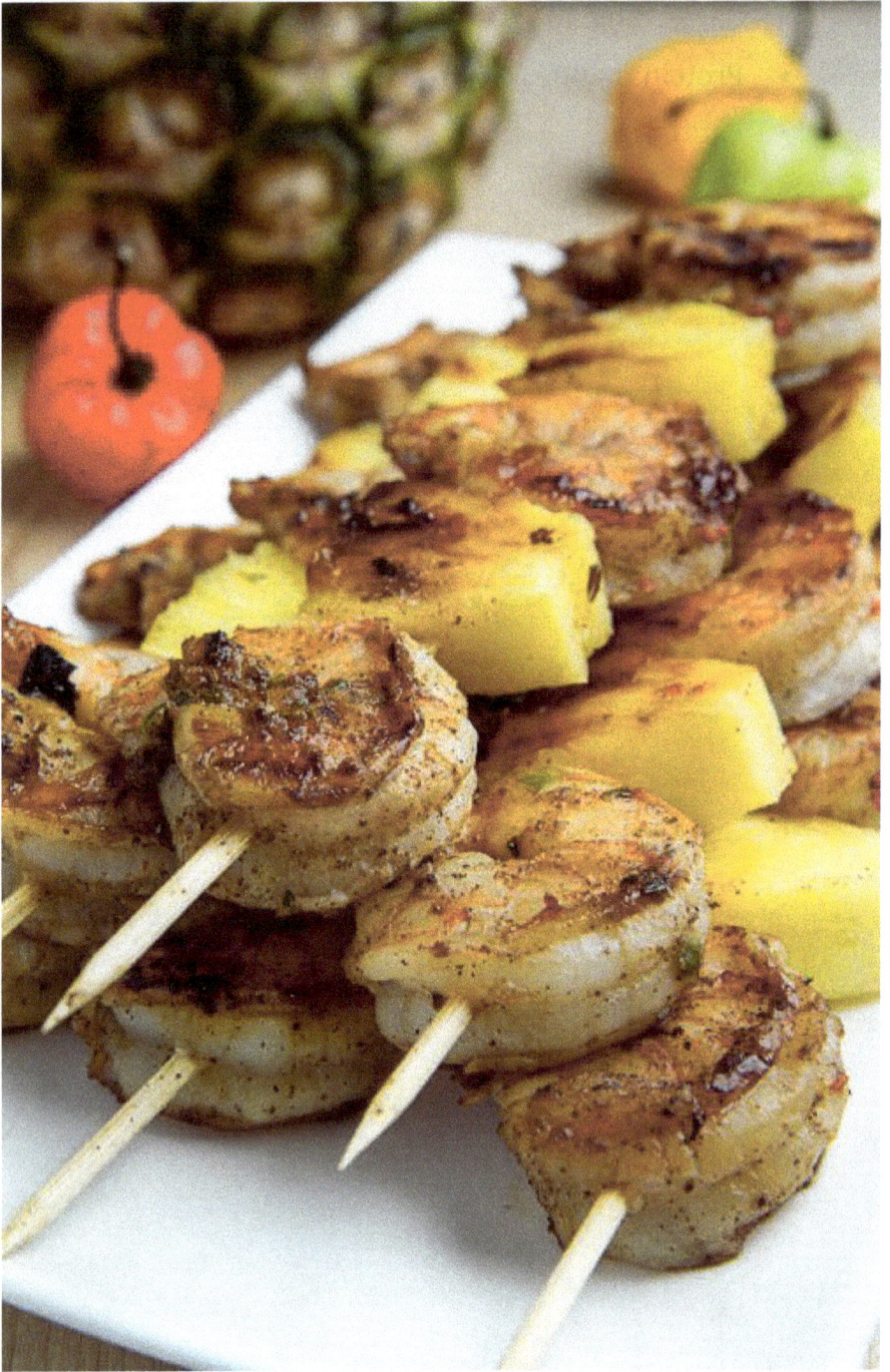

Miso Sauce Over Grilled Salmon

Servings per Recipe: 4

Cooking Time: 16 minutes

Ingredients:

- 1 1/4 pounds skinless salmon fillets, thinly sliced /562.5G

- 1/4 cup yellow miso paste /62.5ML
- 2 tablespoons mirin (Japanese rice wine) /30ML
- 2 teaspoons dashi powder /10G
- 2 teaspoons superfine sugar /10G
- Amaranth leaves (optional), for everyone
- Shichimi togarashi, to serve

Instructions:

1) Add sugar, mirin, dashi powder, and miso in a bowl and mix well.
2) Thread salmon into skewers. Drizzle with miso glaze. Place on skewer rack in the air fryer. If needed, cook in batches.
3) For 8 minutes, cook on 360° F or 183°C . Halfway through cooking time, turnover and drizzle with more miso glaze.
4) Serve and enjoy

Nutrition Information:

- Calories per Serving: 281
- Carbs: 7.6g
- Protein: 39.8g
- Fat: 10.1g

Old Bay 'n Dijon Seasoned Crab Cakes

Servings per Recipe: 2

Cooking Time: 10 minutes

Ingredients:

- ¼ cup chopped green onion /32.5G
- ½ cup panko /65G
- 1 ½ teaspoon old bay seasoning /7.5G
- 1 teaspoon Dijon mustard /5G
- 1 teaspoon Worcestershire sauce /5ML
- 1-pound lump crab meat /450G
- 2 large eggs
- Salt and pepper to taste

Instructions:

1) Preheat the air fryer to 390° F or 199°C .
2) Place the grill pan in the mid-air fryer.
3) In a mixing bowl, combine and stir all Ingredients until properly combined.
4) Form small patties of crab cakes using your hands.
5) Place on the grill pan and cook for 10 Minutes.
6) For even browning flip the crab cakes halfway through cooking time.

Nutrition information:

- Calories per serving: 129
- Carbs: 4.3g
- Protein: 16.2g
- Fat: 5.1g

Orange Roughie with Caesar & Cheese Dressing

Servings per Recipe: 2

Cooking Time: 15

Ingredients:

- 2 orange roughie fillets (4 ounces or /120G each)
- 1/2 cups crushed butter-flavored crackers /65G
- 1/2 cup shredded cheddar cheese /65G
- 1/4 cup creamy Caesar salad dressing /32.5G

Instructions:

1) Sparingly grease the baking pan with oil. Add filet to the bottom of the pan. Sprinkle with dressing and crumbled crackers.
2) Cook for 10 minutes at 390 ° F or 199°C .
3) Sprinkle cheese and allow it to sit for 5 minutes.
4) Serve and enjoy

Nutrition Information:

- Calories per Serving: 341
- Carbs: 5.0g
- Protein: 32.6g
- Fat: 21.1g

Oregano & Cumin Flavored Salmon Grill

Servings per Recipe: 4

Cooking Time: 15

Ingredients:

- 1 1/2 pounds skinless salmon fillet (preferably wild), cut into 1" pieces /675G
- 1 teaspoon ground cumin /5G
- 1 teaspoon kosher salt /5G
- 1/4 teaspoon crushed red pepper flakes /1.25G
- 2 lemons, very thinly sliced into rounds
- 2 tablespoons chopped fresh oregano /30G
- 2 tablespoons essential olive oil /30ML
- 2 teaspoons sesame seeds /10G

Instructions:

1) In a small bowl, combine oregano, sesame seeds, cumin, salt, and pepper flakes. Stir well.
2) Thread salmon and folded lemon slices in a skewer. Brush with oil and dust with seasoning.
3) Place skewers on the air fryer skewer rack.
4) Allow cooking for 5 minutes at 360° F or 183°C . If needed, cook in batches.
5) Serve and enjoy

Nutrition Information:

- Calories per Serving: 313
- Carbs: 2.3g
- Protein: 34.3g
- Fat: 18.5g

Outrageous Crispy Fried Salmon Skin

Serves: 4

Cooking Time: 10 minutes

Ingredients:

- ½ pound salmon skin patted dry /225G
- 4 tablespoons coconut oil /60ML
- Salt and pepper to taste

Instructions:

1) Preheat the air fryer for 5 minutes.
2) In a large mixing bowl, combine all ingredients and mix well.
3) Place inside fryer basket.
4) At 400° For 205°C cook for 10 minutes.
5) Shake the air fryer's basket halfway through cooking time to evenly cook the skin.

Nutrition information:

- Calories per serving: 221
- Carbohydrates: 1.1g
- Protein: 15.2g
- Fat: 16.9g

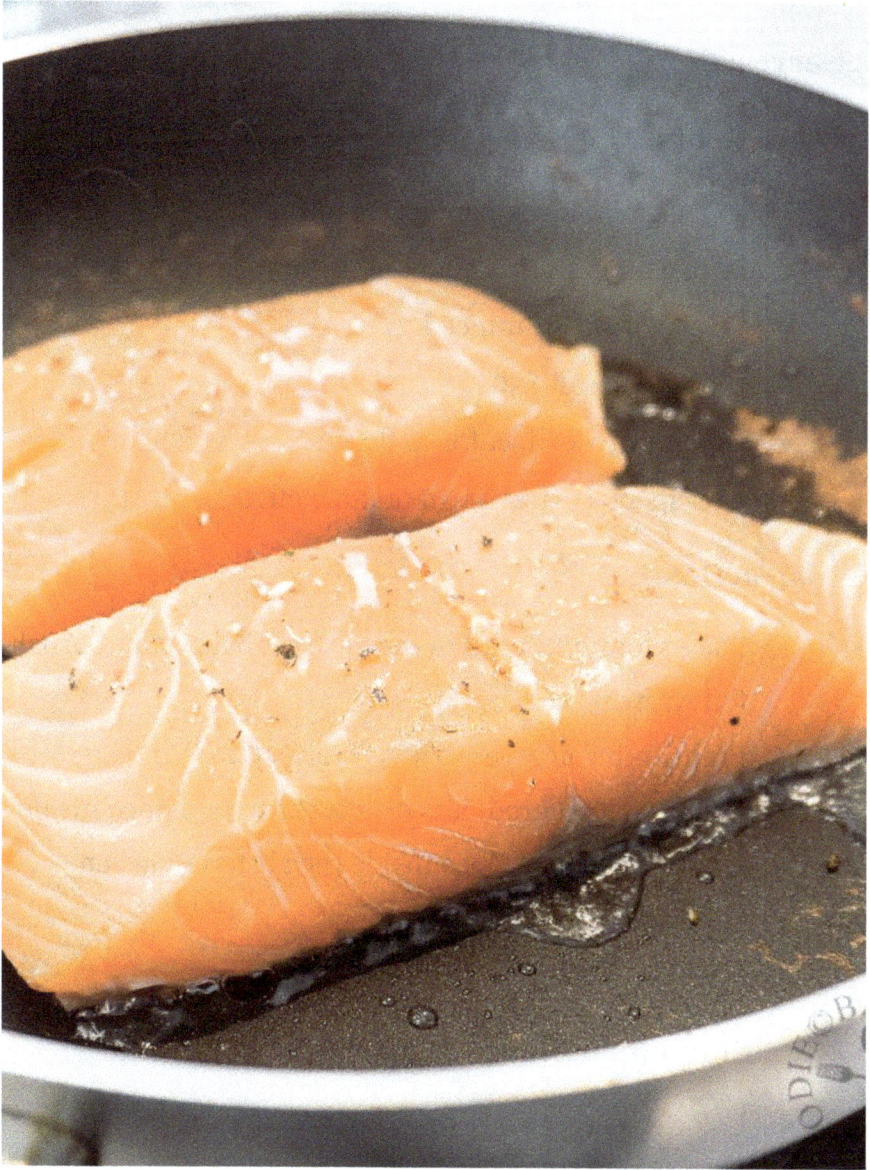

Roasted Broccoli with Salted Garlic

Serves: 6

Ingredients:

- ½ teaspoon black pepper /2.5G
- ½ teaspoon freshly squeezed lemon juice /2.5ML .
- 1 clove of garlic, minced
- 1 teaspoon salt /5G
- 2 heads broccoli, cut into florets
- 2 teaspoons extra virgin organic olive oil /10ML

Instructions

1) Place aluminium foil in the air fryer basket. and brush the foil with oil.
2) Preheat the air fryer to 375° F or 191°C .
3) Combine all ingredients except the lemon juice inside a mixing bowl and place inside the air fryer basket.
4) Cook for 15 minutes.
5) Serve with lemon juice.

Nutrition information:

- Calories per serving: 51
- Carbohydrates: 4.66g
- Protein: 4.86g
- Fat:1.4 g

Roasted Chat-Masala Spiced Broccoli

Servings per Recipe: 2

Cooking Time:15 minutes

Ingredients:

- ¼ teaspoon chat masala /1.25G
- ¼ teaspoons turmeric powder /1.25G
- ½ teaspoon salt /2.5G
- 1 tablespoon chickpea flour /15G
- 2 cups broccoli florets /260G
- 2 tablespoons yogurt /30G

Instructions:

1) Place all ingredients in a bowl, mix well to combine the seasoning with the broccoli florets.
2) Place the broccoli florets in the baking pan and then place the baking pan in the air fryer.
3) Close the air fryer and cook for 15minutes at 330° F or 166°C
4) Shake the basket halfway through cooking time.

Nutrition information:

- Calories per serving:96
- Carbs: 16.8g
- Protein: 7.1g

- Fat:1.3 g

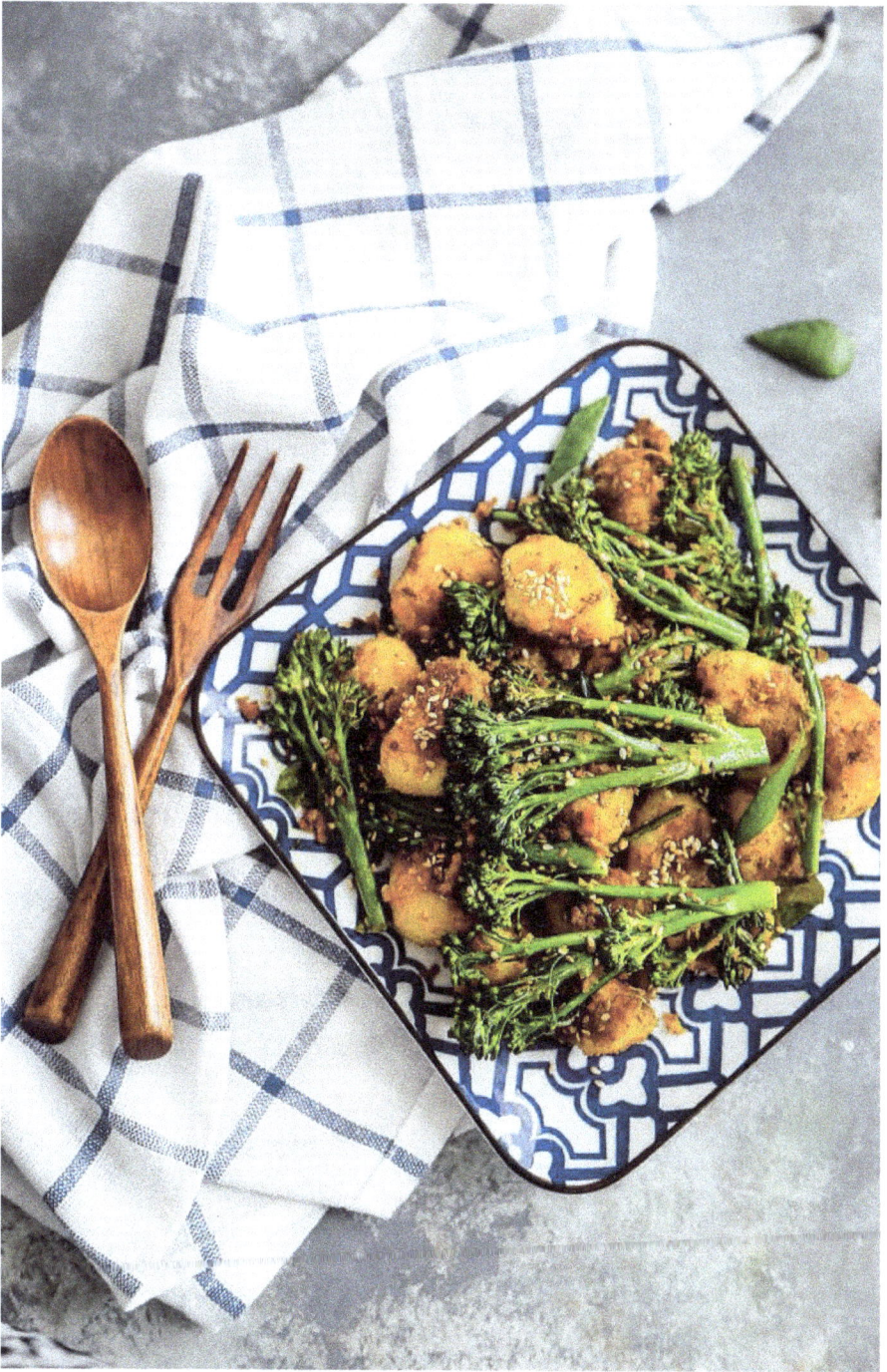

Roasted Mushrooms in Herb-Garlic Oil

Serves: 4

Cooking Time: 25 minutes

Ingredients:

- ½ teaspoon minced garlic /2.5G
- 2 pounds of mushrooms /900G
- 2 teaspoons herbs de Provence /10G
- 3 tablespoons coconut oil /45ML
- Salt and pepper to taste

Instructions:

1) Preheat mid-air fryer for 5 minutes.
2) Place all ingredients in a baking pan that can fit in the mid-air fryer.
3) Mix properly to combine.
4) Place the baking pan in the air fryer.
5) Cook for 25 minutes at 350° F or 177°C .

Nutrition information:

- Calories per serving: 746
- Carbohydrates: 172.2g
- Protein: 12.4g
- Fat: 21.9g

Rosemary Olive-Oil Over Shrooms n Asparagus

Serves: 6

Cooking Time: 15

Ingredients:

- ½ pound fresh mushroom quartered /225G
- 1 bunch of fresh asparagus, trimmed and cleaned
- 2 sprigs of fresh rosemary, minced
- 2 teaspoons essential olive oil /10ML
- salt and pepper to taste

Instructions:

1) Preheat mid-air fryer to 400° F or 205°C .
2) Place the asparagus and mushrooms in the bowl and pour all of those other ingredients.
3) MIx to coat the asparagus and mushrooms.
4) Place inside the air fryer and cook for 15 minutes.

Nutrition information:

- Calories per serving: 149
- Carbohydrates: 29.2g
- Protein: 3.77g
- Fat:1.89 g

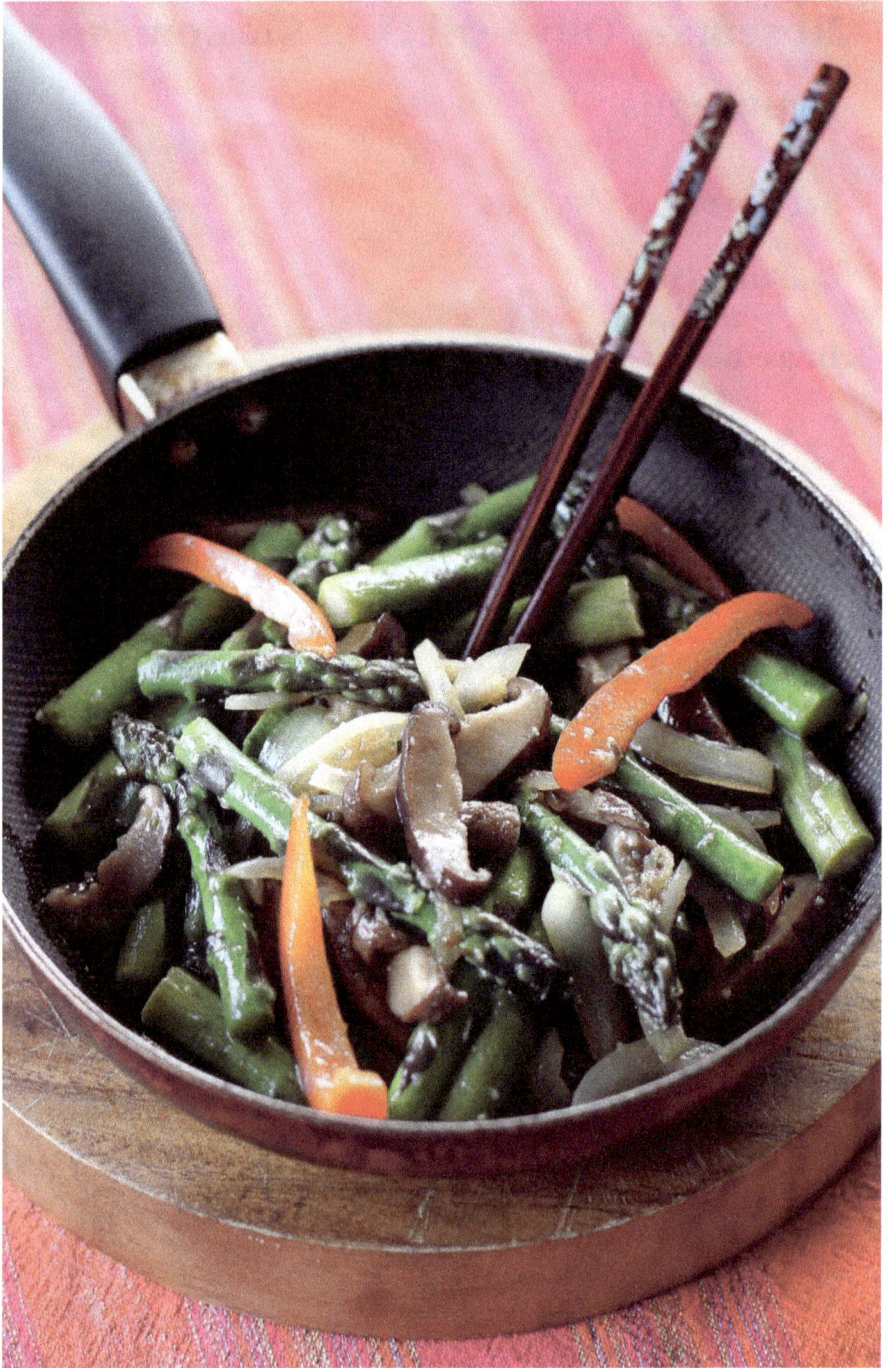

Salted 'n Herbed Potato Packets

Servings per Recipe: 3

Cooking Time: 40 minutes

Ingredients:

- 1 ½ teaspoons seasoning blend /7.5G
- 1 onion, sliced
- 2 large russet potatoes, peeled and sliced
- 2 medium red sweet potatoes, sliced
- 2 tablespoons essential olive oil /30ML
- Salt and pepper to taste

Instructions:

1) Preheat the mid-air fryer to 330° F or 166°C .
2) Place the grill pan in the mid-air fryer.
3) Place all ingredient on a large foil and stir, fold the foil and crumple the sides.
4) Place the foil on the grill pan.
5) Cook for 40 minutes.

Nutrition information:

Calories per serving: 362

Carbs: 68.4g

Protein: 6.3g

Fat: 9.4g

Turmeric and Lemongrass Chicken Roast

Servings per Recipe: 6

Cooking Time: 40 minutes

Ingredients:

- 1 teaspoon turmeric /5G
- 2 lemongrass stalks
- 2 tablespoons fish sauce /30ML
- 3 cloves of garlic, minced
- 3 pounds whole chicken /1150G
- 3 shallots, chopped
- Salt and pepper to taste

Instructions:

1) Place all ingredients in the Ziploc bag and marinate for at least 120 minutes in the fridge.
2) Preheat the air fryer to 390 F or 199°C .
3) Place the grill pan in mid-air fryer.
4) Grill the chicken for 40 minutes and flip over every 10 minutes during grilling.

Nutrition information:

- Calories per serving: 495
- Carbs: 49.1g

- Protein: 38.5g;
- Fat: 16.1g

Apple Pie in Air Fryer

Servings per Recipe: 4

Cooking Time: 35 minutes

Ingredients:

- ½ teaspoon vanilla flavoring /2.5ML
- 1 beaten egg
- 1 large apple, chopped
- 1 Pillsbury Refrigerator pie crust
- 1 tablespoon butter /15G
- 1 tablespoon ground cinnamon /15G
- 1 tablespoon raw sugar /15G
- 2 tablespoon sugar /15G
- 2 teaspoons fresh lemon juice /10ML
- Baking spray

Instructions:

1) Using a cooking spray grease lightly the baking pan of an air fryer. Spread pie crust in the pan evenly.
2) Mix vanilla, sugar, cinnamon, lemon juice, and apples in a bowl. Pour this mixture on top of the pie crust. Add apples with butter slice on top too.
3) Cover using the remaining pie crust. Pierce the top of the pie with a knife.

4) Spread beaten eggs on top of the crust and sprinkle with sugar.
5) Cover with foil.
6) Cook at 390° F or 199°C for 25 minutes.
7) Remove foil and cook for an additional 10 minutes at 330° F or 166°C or until tops are brown.
8) Serve and enjoy.

Nutrition Information:

- Calories per Serving: 372
- Carbs: 44.7g
- Protein: 4.2g
- Fat: 19.6g

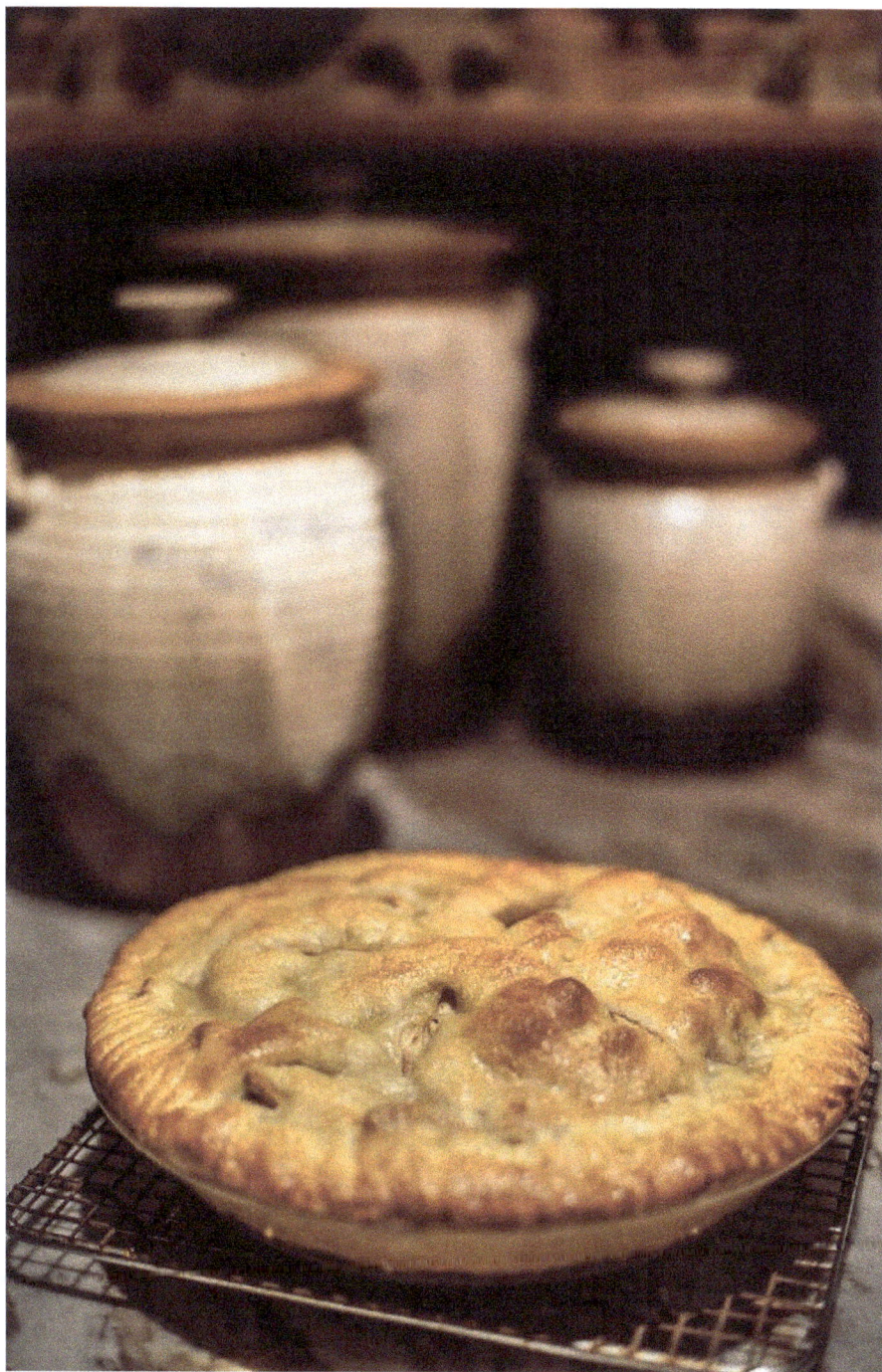

Apple-Toffee Upside-Down Cake

Serves: 9

Cooking Time: 30 Minutes

Ingredients

- ¼ cup almond butter /32.5G
- ¼ cup sunflower oil /62.5ML
- ½ cup walnuts, chopped /65G
- ¾ cup + 3 tablespoon coconut sugar /138G
- ¾ cup water /188ML
- 1 ½ teaspoon mixed spice /7.5G
- 1 cup plain flour /130G
- 1 lemon, zest
- 1 teaspoon baking soda /5G
- 1 teaspoon vinegar /5ML
- 3 baking apples, cored and sliced

Instructions:

1) Preheat air fryer to 390° F or 199°C .
2) Melt the almond butter and 3 tablespoons of sugar in a pan. Pour the mixture into the baking dish. Arrange the slices of apples on top. Set aside.
3) Add flour, ¾ cup sugar, and baking soda. Add the mixed spice.

4) Mix the oil, water, vinegar, and lemon zest. Add chopped walnuts and stir.

5) Combine both wet ingredients and dry ingredients. Mix well until well combined.

6) Place apple slices in the pan.

7) Bake for 30 minutes or place a toothpick in the middle of the pie if it comes out clean then the pie is cooked.

Nutrition information:

- Calories per serving: 335
- Carbohydrates: 39.6g
- Protein: 3.8g
- Fat: 17.9g

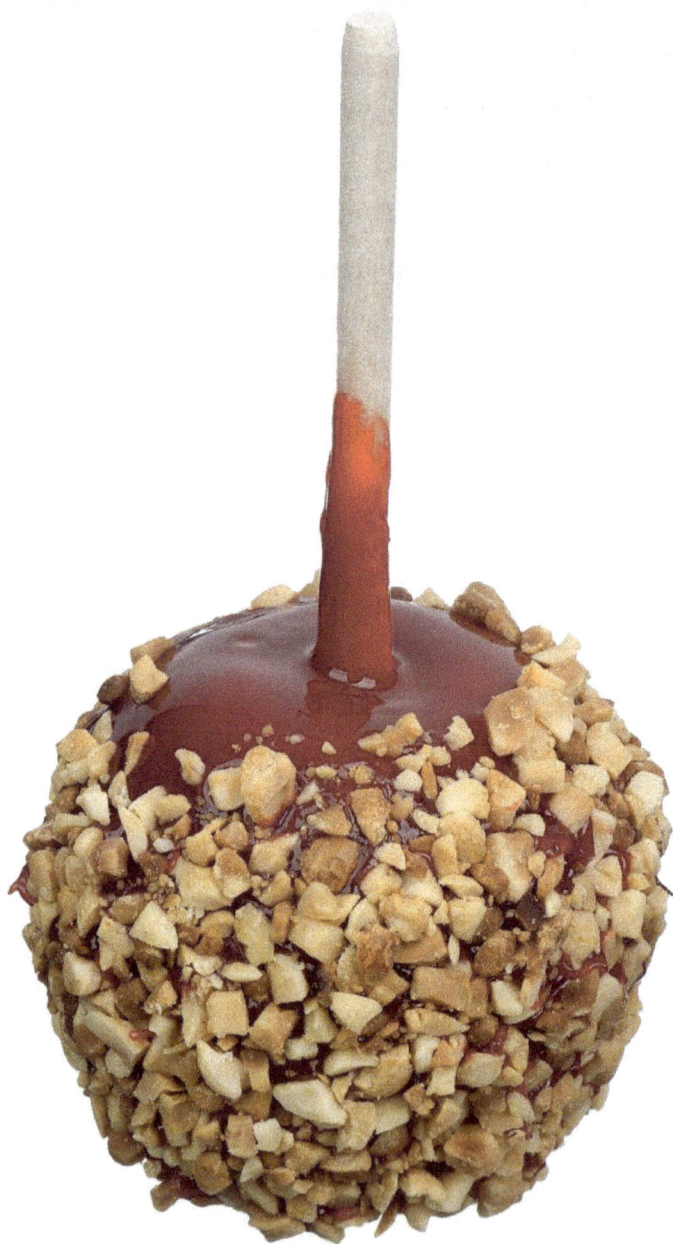

Banana-Choco Brownies

Serves: 12

Cooking Time: 30 Minutes

Ingredients:

- 2 cups almond flour /260G
- 2 teaspoons baking powder /10G
- ½ teaspoon baking powder /2.5G
- ½ teaspoon baking soda /2.5G
- ½ teaspoon salt /2.5G
- 1 over-ripe banana
- 3 large eggs
- ½ teaspoon stevia powder /2.5G
- ¼ cup coconut oil /62.5ML
- 1 tablespoon vinegar /15ML
- 1/3 cup almond flour /43G
- 1/3 cup hot chocolate mix /43G

Instructions:

1) Preheat the air fryer for 5 minutes.
2) Blend all ingredients.
3) Pour the mixture into a baking dish.
4) Place in the air fryer basket and cook for 30 minutes at 350° F or 177°C or if a toothpick inserted in the middle comes out clean.

Nutrition information:

- Calories per serving: 75
- Carbohydrates: 2.1g
- Protein: 1.7g
- Fat: 6.6g

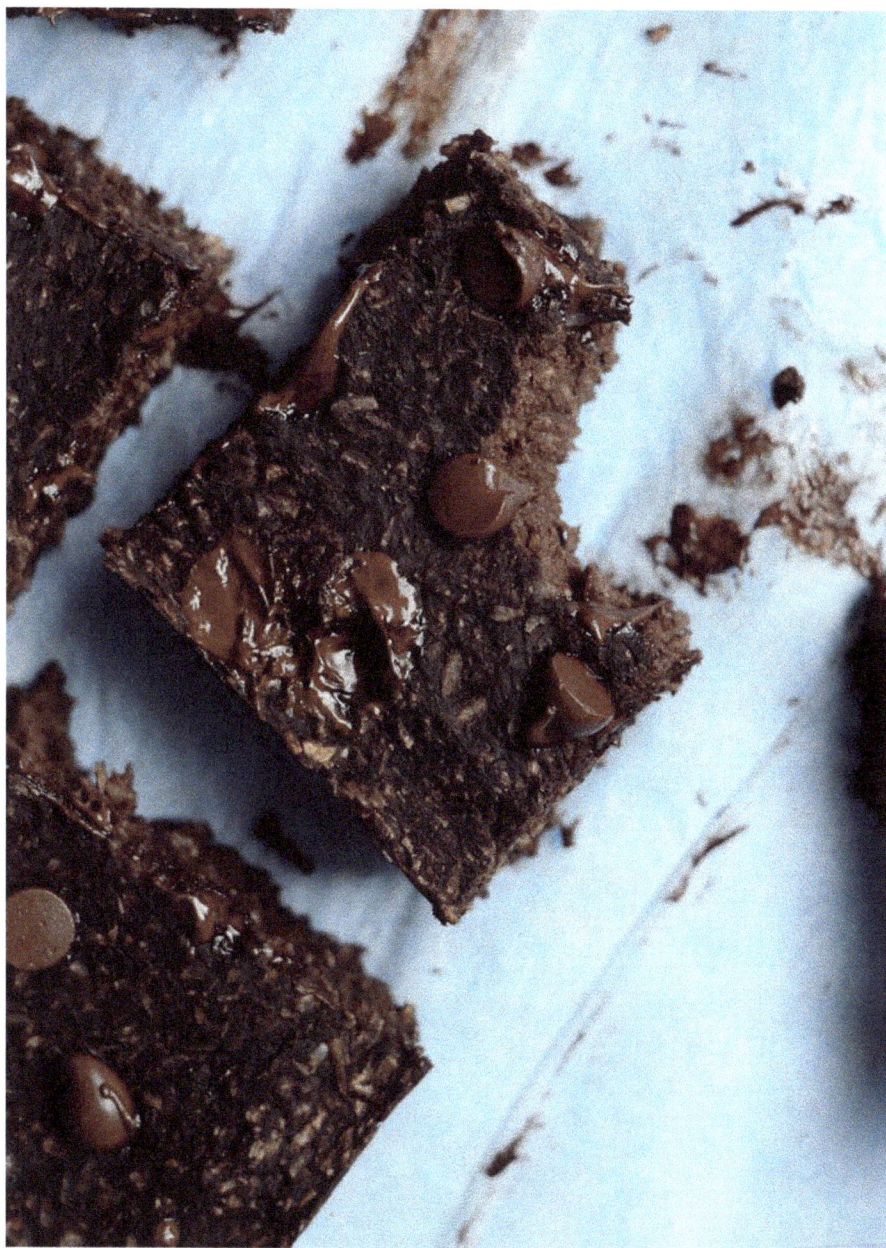

www.ingramcontent.com/pod-product-compliance
Lightning Source LLC
Chambersburg PA
CBHW050747030426
42336CB00012B/1695